THE
Tasmania Pantry Cookbook 2

Simple and delicious recipes inspired by Tasmanian growers and producers

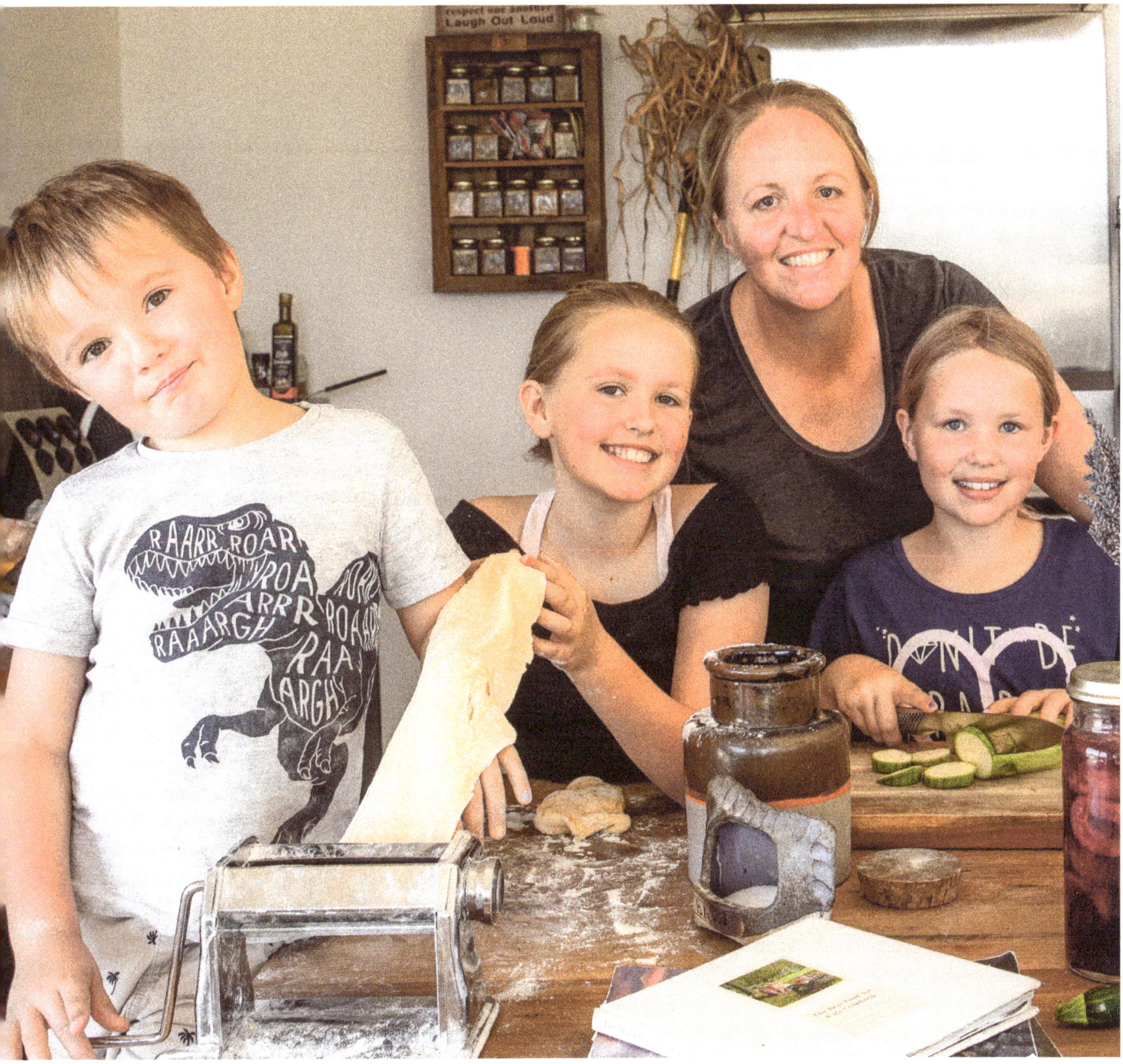

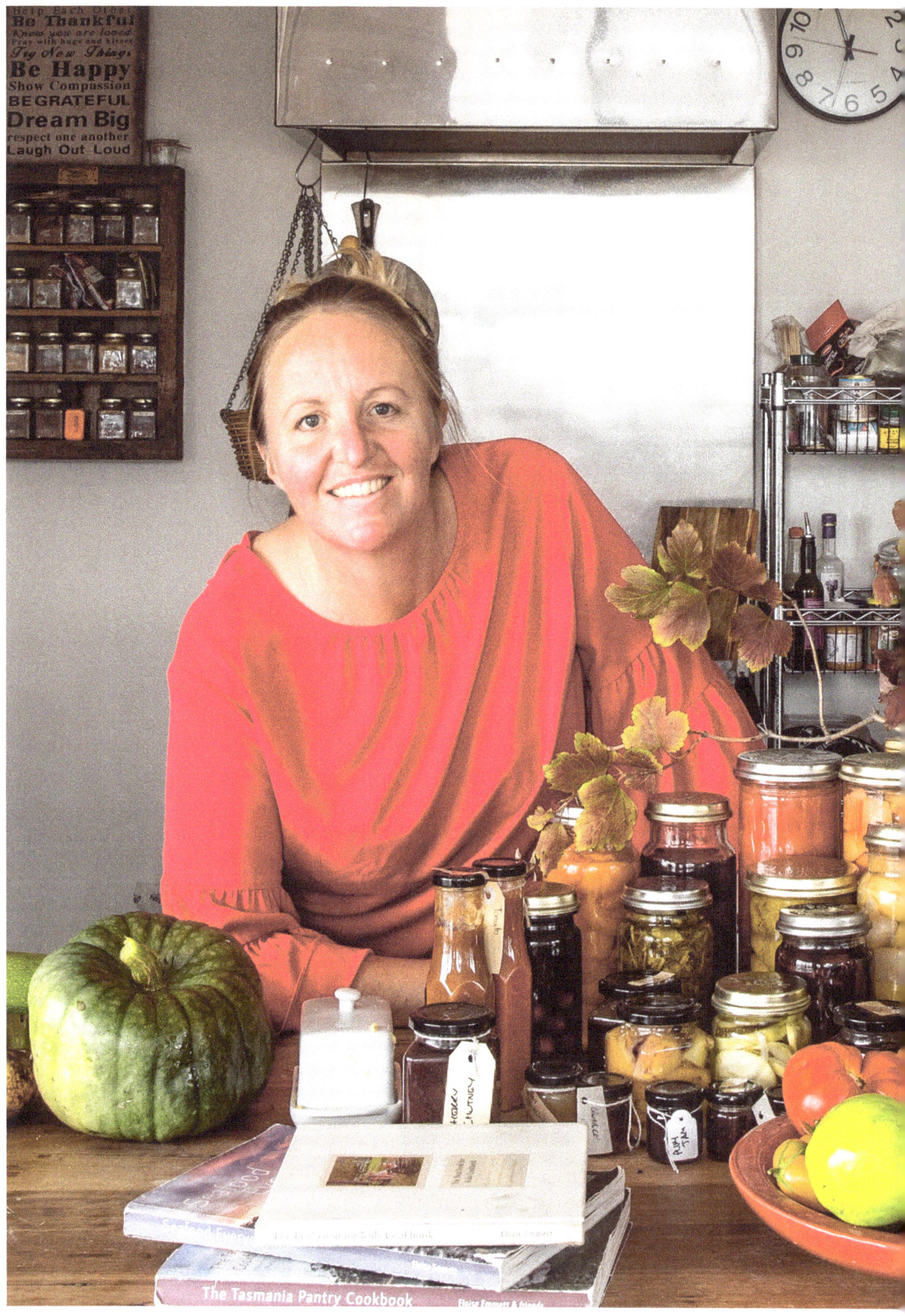

The Tasmania Pantry Cookbook 2

Living in Tasmania with an abundance of fresh fruit and veggies, spacious pastures for high quality meat, excellent quality extra virgin olive oil and being surrounded by the ocean for seafood, it is easy to follow a Mediterranean-ish style diet.

Food fads come and go, all the while pushing a diet culture, creating harm to people's physical and mental health and of course, their body image. The Mediterranean style of eating is not a weight-loss diet, rather a healthy eating plan, which has been scientifically proven to improve mental health as well as many other health ailments.

The recent research on gut health whilst following a Mediterranean style diet is quite mind blowing. The crux of the diet is to eat around 1 kilo of fruit and vegetables per day. This may sound like a lot, but when you consider an apple may weigh 150 grams it doesn't take that long to add up. I estimate that we need roughly 35 kilos of fruit and vegetables per week, for a family of five. Even in the middle of winter when we are getting barely anything from our own garden, our fruit and vegetable bill is rarely over $100 for the week.

In this insane year of 2020, looking after yourself and maintaining good health has never been more important. Rather than focusing on limiting, counting or restricting foods, instead I encourage my family to enjoy a wide variety of delicious plants.

The research on gut health and the links to improvements in mental health fascinates me. To think a few small simple adjustments to the diet - such as slowing down and chewing to help digestion, adding a few tablespoons of fermented foods a day, eating at least 30 different plants a week, enjoying meals with family and friends - could have such positive results on mental as well as physical health. Why wouldn't we all at least try? Sadly and quite shockingly, in Tasmania up to 96 percent of people in some age groups do not eat enough fruit and veggies each day.

Food marketing will try to convince us that cooking is hard and time consuming, but I am here to tell you it is not. It is also the most affordable and healthiest way to feed your family as you know exactly what you are eating. Large food companies are not concerned about the health of your family, so a lot of packet food is full of cheap and nasty oils and produce.

I am a realist - as much as I love using my own home-grown food and sourcing it locally, we happily use Australian tinned tomatoes when tomatoes are not in season or my own preserved supply has run out. I just do the best I can. I am so grateful for farmers - I love being in my garden - but we would literally starve if we had to eat only out of our garden through winter in Tasmania! Maybe one day!

As a busy mum of three young children I do not find it hard, time-consuming, or expensive at all to organise our family to eat our veggies every day. It can be easy to get stuck in a rut with meals, especially in the middle of winter in Tasmania, so I hope this book can bring a little inspiration to your family table for weekdays and special occasions.

Eloise Emmett 2020

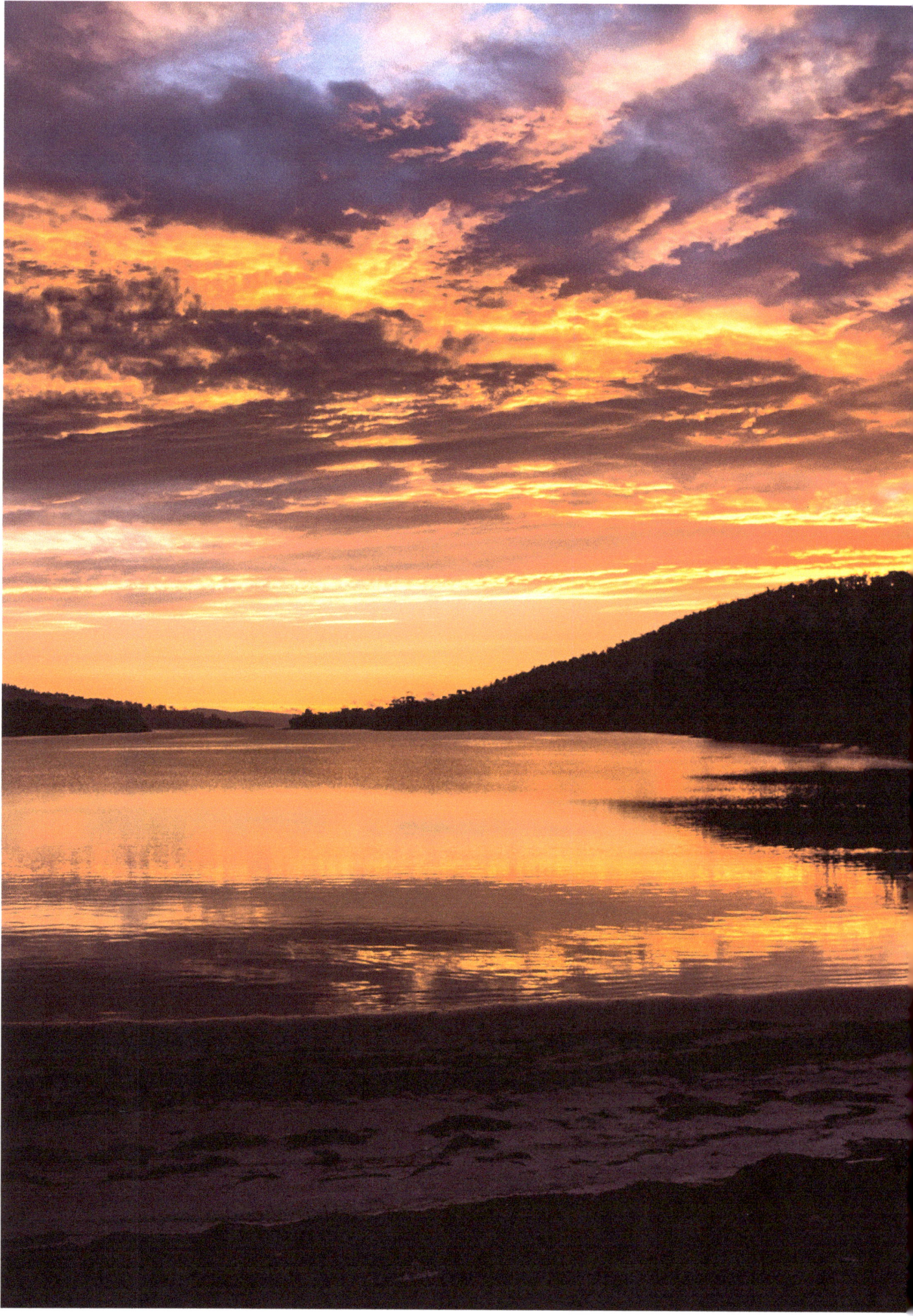

Acknowledgements

Thanks to Kylie Berry, Stokely 9 Design, for the beautiful design and support with the creation of this book.

Thanks to the generous sponsors as without them, this book would be not be possible. Thanks for their enthusiasm and ease to work with and of course the beautiful products they produce for me to enjoy creating recipes with.

Fiona	Freshfield Grove
Lisa	Campo De Flori
Tess, Judy and Will	Mures Tasmania
Mark and Beck	Lost Pipin Cider
Caroline and Ben	Tassal
Sally	Lenah Game Meats
Fred	Bream Creek Vineyard
Jackie	Puddleduck Vineyard
Carley	Van Diemens Land Creamery
Cathy	TasFoods
Julie	Freycinet Marine Farm
Corrine and Chris	Wild Pepper Isle
Liz	Summerlea Farm
Leanne	Cameron of Tasmania Oyster Farm
	Christmas Hill Raspberry Farm
	Hill Street Home

Thanks to my family, my husband Brendan and children Maggie, Stephanie and Oscar who are happy to pop on a good shirt for a photo and enjoy all the foods.

Thanks to my workshop, event and dinner guests at Little Norfolk Bay Events and Chalets, who taste all the recipes and inspire me to create new dishes.

Thanks to Arwen Genge and Natalie Jones for all the cooking for the photos, recipe testing and editing.

Thanks to the amazing tableware creators in Tasmania for making my images look so pretty with your works of art. Lisa Britzman, Bronwyn Clarke, Ben and Peta Richardson, Ian Claire, Sallee Warner, Yolanda Zarins, Sarah Webb, Cate Foley-Burke and Lisa West work appears frequently in this book.

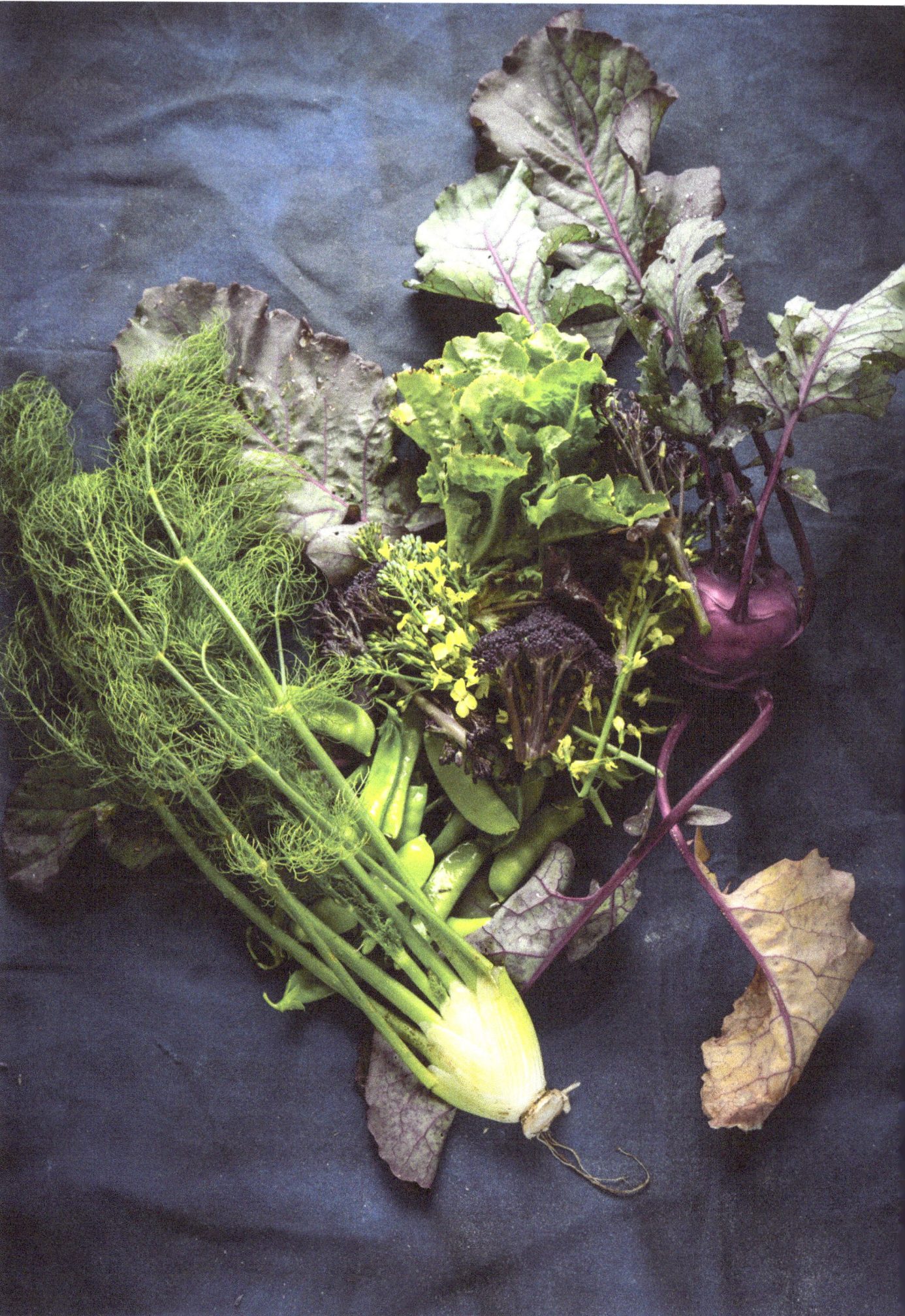

Handy hints and kitchen tips

BREAD BAKING

In the bread recipes, I add the water measurement in a range, depending on the flour you are using.

The humidity and freshness of the flour you may need a little more water. A wetter dough will result in a light bread. Although not time consuming, you do need time to make good bread, rushing and not allowing it to rise enough will only give you a solid not well risen bread.

THRIFTY COOKING

My mum is a great one for using up what you have in the pantry and fridge. I guess she would be fashionable now with the No Waste Movement! A lot of the recipes in this book can be used as a guide and you can make your own variation, make sure you share your variations on my social media as it might just inspire another person to cook something from their cupboard or refrigerator!

COOKING MEAT

When cooking meat, it will cook slowly until the fat heats up (around rare) and then cook quickly. For example, a scotch fillet may take 10 minutes to reach rare when cooking on the barbeque and then within two minutes it is overcooked. Your meat and poultry needs to be rested for around the same time as it is cooked, so always under cook before resting.

PRESENTATION

If you want your food to look good then an investment in some gorgeous handmade ceramics is the best start. My number one food styling tip is to start with a beautiful plate.

KEEP IT SIMPLE

I simplify my recipes for the home kitchen. I try not to use exotic ingredients that may only be used for a one-off recipe. I imagine myself in my car needing to drive to a specialty food store for one particular ingredient, find a park, remove the 3 kids from the car. Do I actually NEED that ingredient, or could I substitute it and still get a delicious result? Rotating stock in the pantry is always important in the home or commercial kitchen. It is not just your money sitting on the shelf, things like flours, grains and nuts actually do go stale, so using them as quickly as possible is always good. Do we really need that fancy specialty flour and have 6 different bags of flour open or would the one bread or plain flour do? I would prefer to purchase an economical bulk bag and empty it relatively quickly. When we simplify the process we are likely to do it more.

GARLIC

My 2019 garlic harvest had a few black spots on it as it was harvested after heavy rain. Worried it would rot when hanging to store I washed and puréed the garlic whole with the skin and scapes and then vacuum packed it onto 500 gram packs. These packs when defrosted are then put into a jar and covered with extra virgin olive ready for cooking. All my workshop guests love this tip, the garlic is strong in flavour and we have less waste from rot and saving the skins and scapes. I will be doing this all the time from now on.

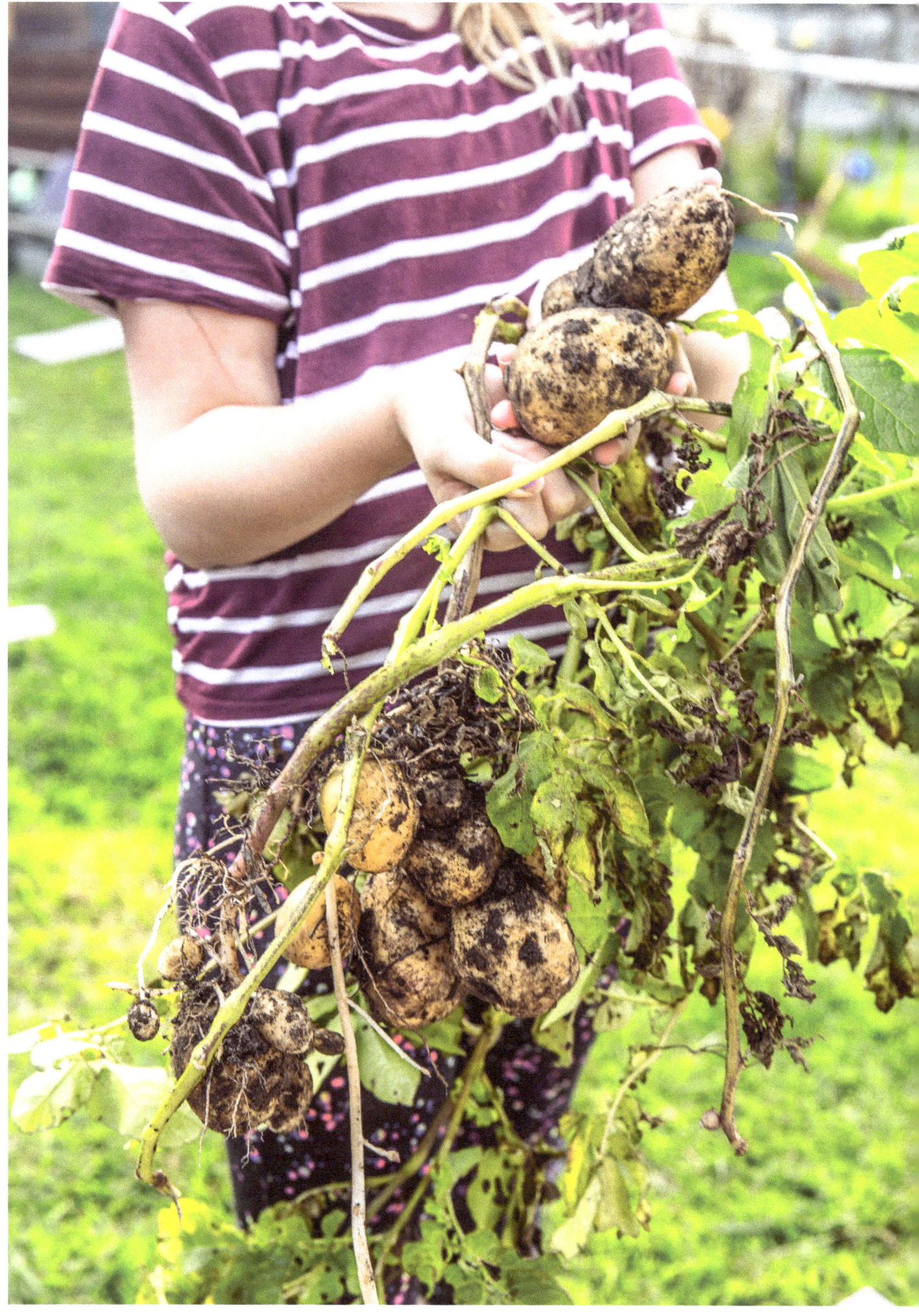

EXTRA VIRGIN OLIVE OIL

Along with salt and pepper, extra virgin olive oil is essential to season our food and it has many health benefits, unlike other fats and oils that can be bad for us. A 'robust' extra virgin olive oil is herbaceous and green, and has a strong flavour with a peppery and pungent finish. There are many other flavours and differences that can be identified between the robust oils. A mild or sometimes referred to as 'delicate' olive oil, has a ripe fruit flavour and milder in pepper and pungency again many other flavours can be identified. The oil, generally, should complement the product you are cooking with, but sometimes contrast is good too. Creamy sweet feta cheese and a robust oil to marinate it in is an example of when the contrast is good.

STOCK

A good stock is handy for the base of a tasty sauce, soup and many other meals. It is also a great way to avoid waste in your kitchen. The peelings and trimmings from aromatic vegetables such as carrots, leeks, celery, onions and herbs can be popped into a bag in the freezer to access easily when making your stocks, reserving the whole vegetable for consumption in the dish. There is more information on my website on how I easily make stocks in my home kitchen with my slow cooker.

REDUCE WASTE

Reducing food waste is both economically and environmentally responsible. To reduce kitchen waste store your food well and use it within the appropriate recommended time period. Washing and spinning lettuces, herbs and other greens and storing in a container in the fridge will maintain freshness. Make a soup out of left over veggies in the fridge at the end of week. Only buying what you are planning to use, eating seasonally and locally will always be more economical.

CHILDREN

Get your kids in the kitchen when they are young. Obviously, I wouldn't let my toddler in the kitchen with

hot fat on the stove bubbling away for deep frying, but they can't do that much damage with a peeler! Peeling veggies, rolling pasta, helping knead dough, the kids can come in and help with many different jobs while you are cooking. The aim being that they should be able to prepare and cook basic meals with supervision around the age of 10. If you want your kids to eat well and enjoy veggies, then have them in the kitchen with you.
They will most likely eat the veggies off the bench whilst you are cooking!

"Starting with excellent quality ingredients is the key to delicious food."

Crayfish Bisque

SERVES 4

In this recipe, we are serving the bisque as a soup with the crayfish meat and a drizzle (OK dump!) of lemon agrumato. We are using the whole fish but you could just use the shell from another fish you have cooked. This bisque makes a fancy entrée or a nice simple lunch. You can also use a thickened bisque as a beautiful sauce for steamed or baked fish or other seafood such as oysters, or use the bisque in a seafood risotto, seafood stew or for pasta. So, if you make more than you need you can pop it in the freezer for a quick meal or sauce for another meal on another day.

A little hot No Waste Tip here - In all my stock making I recommend replacing the onion, leek and carrot with the trimmings of those veggies. The idea is to collect and freeze the off-cuts of these common ingredients, ready to use for a variety of stock recipes. I rarely use an actual whole vegetable for the stock, saving them for the dish that will actually be consumed. For more information on stock making, see my website www.eloiseemmett.com.

1 cooked crayfish

1 onion

1 leek white

1 carrot

1 clove garlic

1 bay leaf

2 sprigs thyme

1 splash robust extra virgin olive oil

1 tablespoon butter

1 teaspoon tarragon

60 grams plain flour

800ml water

400 grams tomato

salt and pepper

2 tablespoons lemon agrumato

Remove the meat from the crayfish. Crush the shell in a heavy based pot with a meat mallet and add the roughly chopped onion, leek, carrot, garlic and tarragon. Sauté with the oil and butter for about 4 minutes over a low heat until the vegetables have softened.

Add the flour and continue cooking for around 5 minutes. Add the water, tomato, salt and pepper and simmer for 30 minutes. Leave to cool and infuse for a few hours and then strain the stock from the shell and stock vegetables and discard the shell and vegetables.

Purée the stock and bring back to a gentle simmer. Chop the crayfish into a rough 1cm dice and add the crayfish and simmer for 2 minutes, or until the fish is just cooked. Season and serve with crusty bread and drizzled with lemon agrumato.

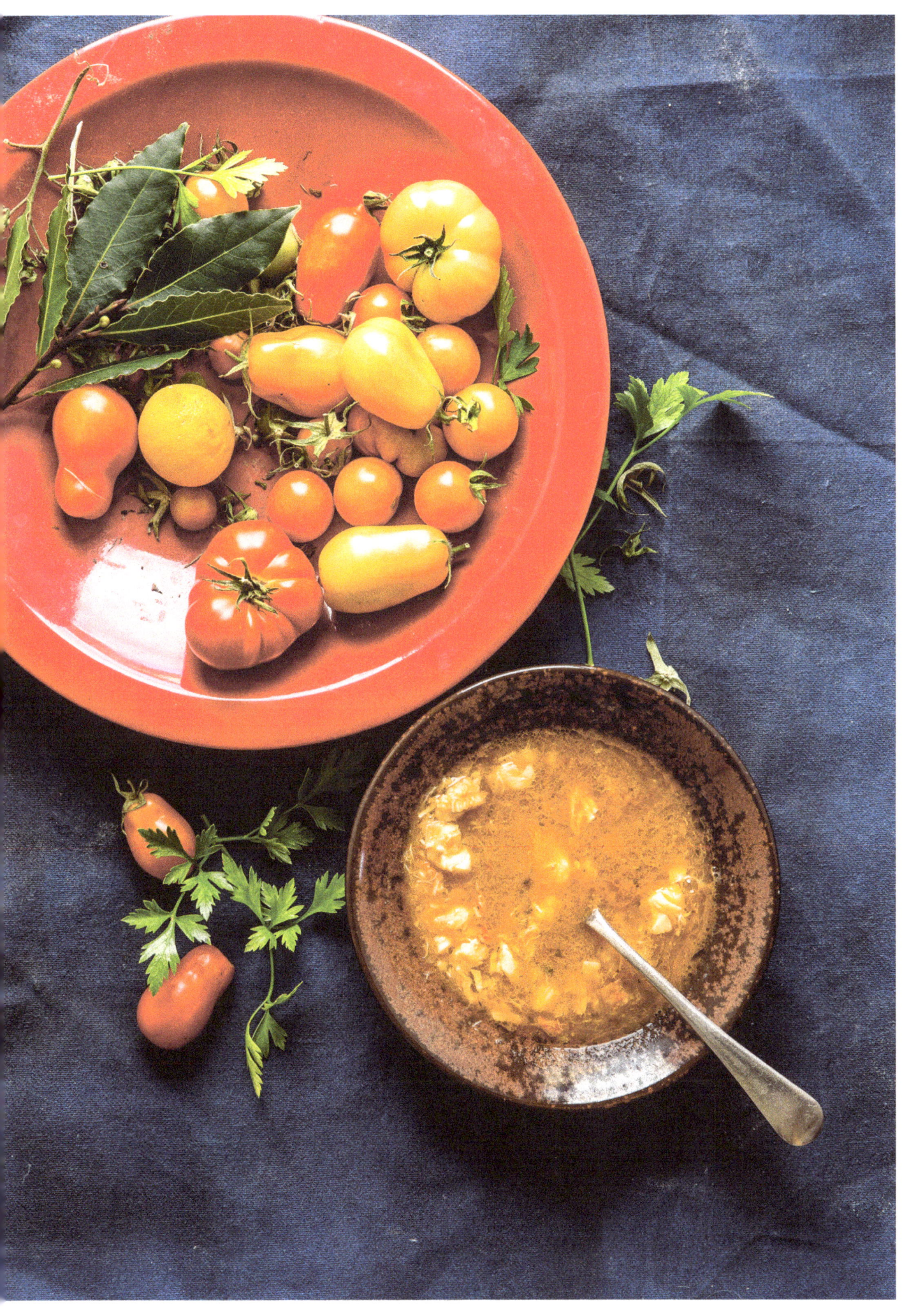

Green Tomato and Lentil Soup

SERVES 4

I created this soup after planting my tomatoes way too late one year. There is only so much green tomato pickle and chutney a person can make! Serve this delicious soup with a spoonful of natural yogurt and some flat bread. When I have mountains of green tomatoes from my garden, I will freeze them in 700 gram portions to make this soup during the winter.

1 brown onion

2 medium carrots

2 stalks celery

2 cloves garlic

robust extra virgin olive oil

½ teaspoon cumin

½ teaspoon garam marsala

½ teaspoon ground coriander seed

¼ teaspoon chilli

¼ teaspoon dry ginger

700 grams green tomatoes

150 grams red lentils

700ml chicken or vegetable stock

salt and pepper

OPTIONAL TO SERVE

yogurt

flat breads

Peel and dice the onion, carrot, celery and crush garlic. Heat a good dash of oil in a large heavy based pan and add the onion, carrot, celery, cumin, garlic, garam masala, coriander, chilli and ginger to the pan and sauté for 3 or 4 minutes, until the vegetables are soft and the spices aromatic.

Add the chopped tomatoes, lentils and stock to the pot and simmer for 30 minutes. Purée if you prefer a smooth soup.

Season with salt and pepper and serve.

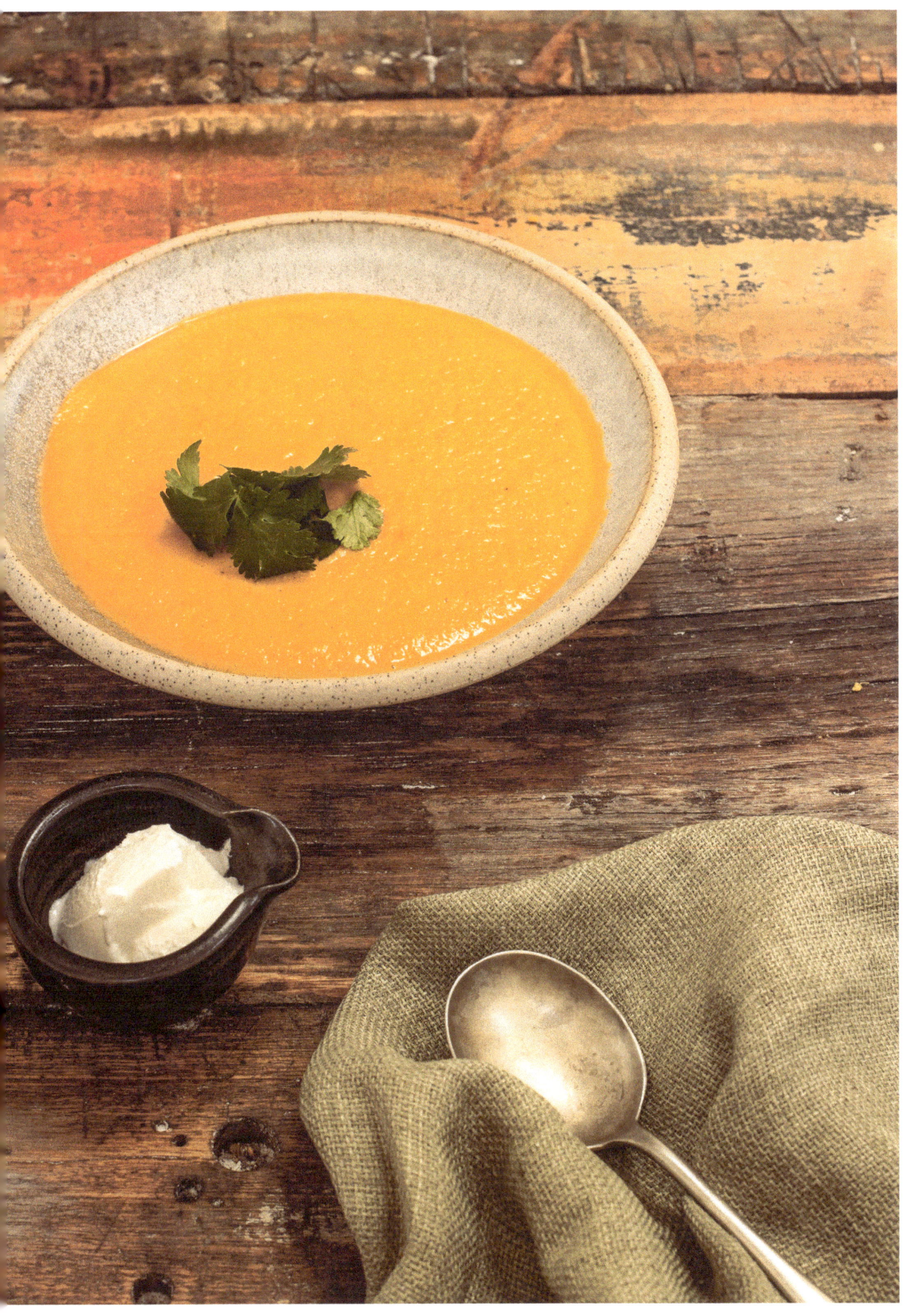

Fruit Loaf

MAKES AROUND 18 SLICES

It has taken quite a few loaves to perfect this recipe. I use my thermocooker to knead my bread dough but you can use any mixer or knead by hand on the bench if you want an arm work out. Shaping your dough correctly is an important step in bread making process. Rolling the dough out flat and then rolling it up into a tight log before leaving it to rise again will give the loaf structure.

We are spoilt for choice in Tasmania with beautiful honey to use in this loaf; the honey adds a beautiful flavour to the bread. This bread, toasted and simply lathered with butter, is a regular breakfast in our house. I will bake the loaf on the weekend and freeze the slices. My daughter Stephanie loves her morning fruit toast topped with cinnamon, sliced apple and ricotta.

500 grams plain flour

1 teaspoon salt

15 grams brown sugar

20 grams honey

2 teaspoons mixed spice

1 teaspoon cinnamon

2 teaspoons dry yeast

30 grams butter

1 tablespoon bread improver

300ml - 320ml lukewarm water

130 grams dried fruit (sultanas, currants, raisins, cherries, cranberries)

Put all the ingredients apart from the dried fruit into the thermocooker bowl and knead for 2 minutes. Alternatively, mix the ingredients in a bowl to form a dough and knead the dough on a floured bench for around 15 minutes to form a smooth dough.

Add the fruit and knead for another 2 minutes. Cover the dough and leave to rise in a warm place until it has doubled in size.

Shape the dough into a ball and then roll out flat on a floured bench with a rolling pin. Starting with one side of the dough, roll the dough up into a tight sausage and place on a baking tray.

Place the loaf in a warm spot until it has doubled in size. Bake in a hot 220°C oven for around 20 minutes and then turn the oven down to 190°C to finish cooking for around 10 minutes.

The loaf should be golden brown and cooked through, and should sound hollow when knocked with your knuckles.

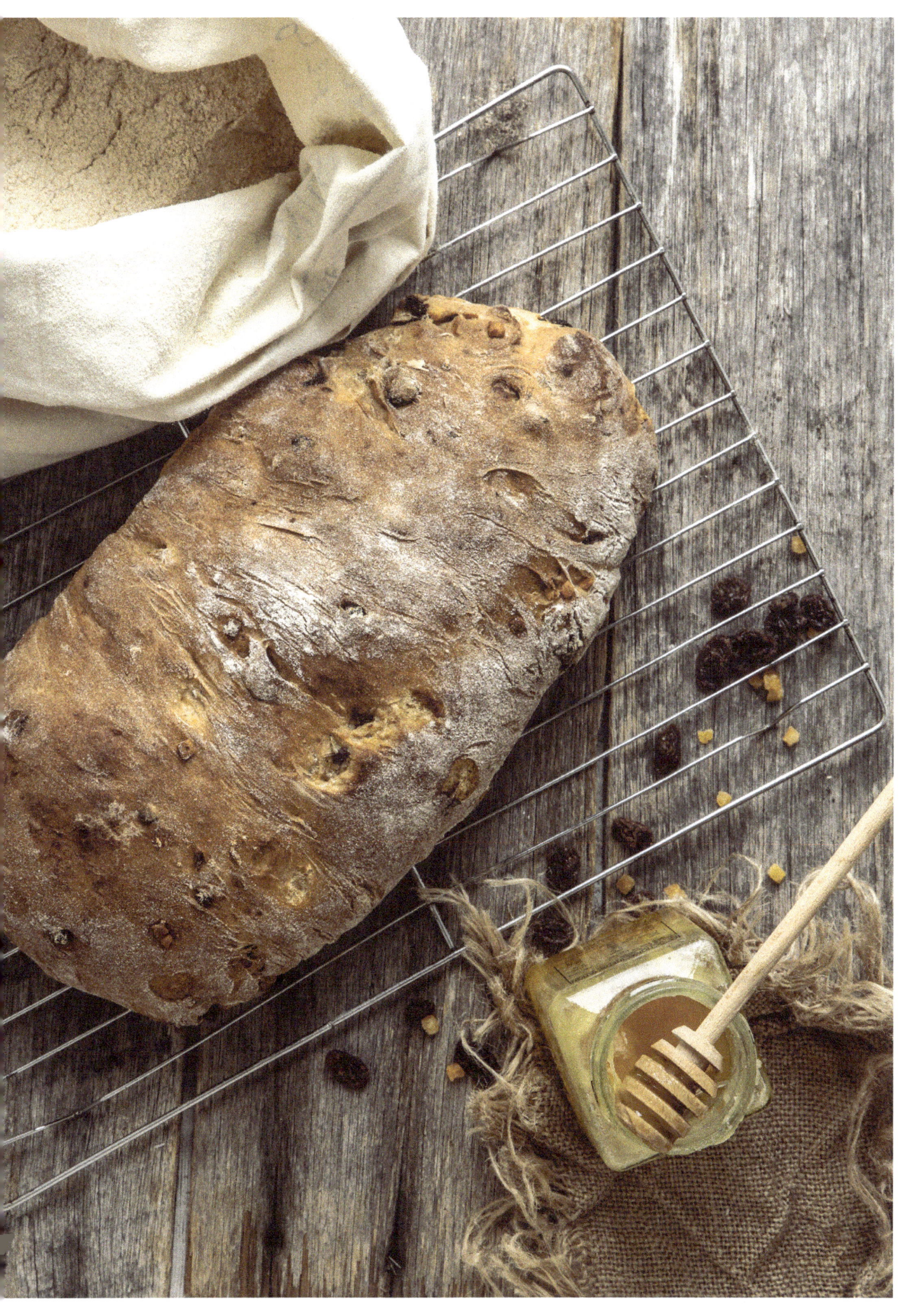

Quail with a Quinoa, Citrus and Herb Salad

SERVES 4

Quail from Rannoch Farm is always a great choice, it's not at all hard to cook and super easy to do on the barbeque. Bruce, Rannoch Farm owner, and I have a difference of opinion on how long to cook the little boned butterflied birds. I don't mind them slightly pink whereas Bruce's recipe would add another 5 minutes cooking time. If cooking them is not something you feel comfortable doing, or you have a lot of guests to feed and you don't want the pressure, then simply purchase the smoked and ready to serve quail, which is an exceptional product! This recipe is extremely popular with my dining guests at Little Norfolk Bay Events and Chalets.

We all want to eat quinoa – it is good for us and grown in Tasmania - but when using it as a replacement for rice it can be the less appetising option. However, quinoa has certainly found its place in my salads, especially light and fruity salads like this one.

1 lemon

2 oranges

1 small clove garlic

8 large mint leaves

4 small silver-beet leaves (or spinach or lettuce)

2 tablespoons parsley

2 tablespoons robust extra virgin olive oil

pepper

sea salt

4 Rannoch Farm Quail, boned and butterflied

1 cup cooked quinoa (I use Kindred Organics brand) cooked to the packet directions and cooled.

To make the salad, segment the oranges and lemons or simply peel the fruit and divide the flesh up, depending on how fancy you are feeling.

Mix in the cooked quinoa crushed garlic clove, sliced mint and parsley leaves and silver-beet. Dress with one tablespoon of the olive oil and a good pinch of cracked black pepper and sea salt.

To cook the quail, heat a heavy based pan to a medium high heat and add the remaining oil. Add the quail skin side down, turn once or twice mostly skin side down for about 6 minutes until the birds are just cooked through.

Serve the birds hot with the salad.

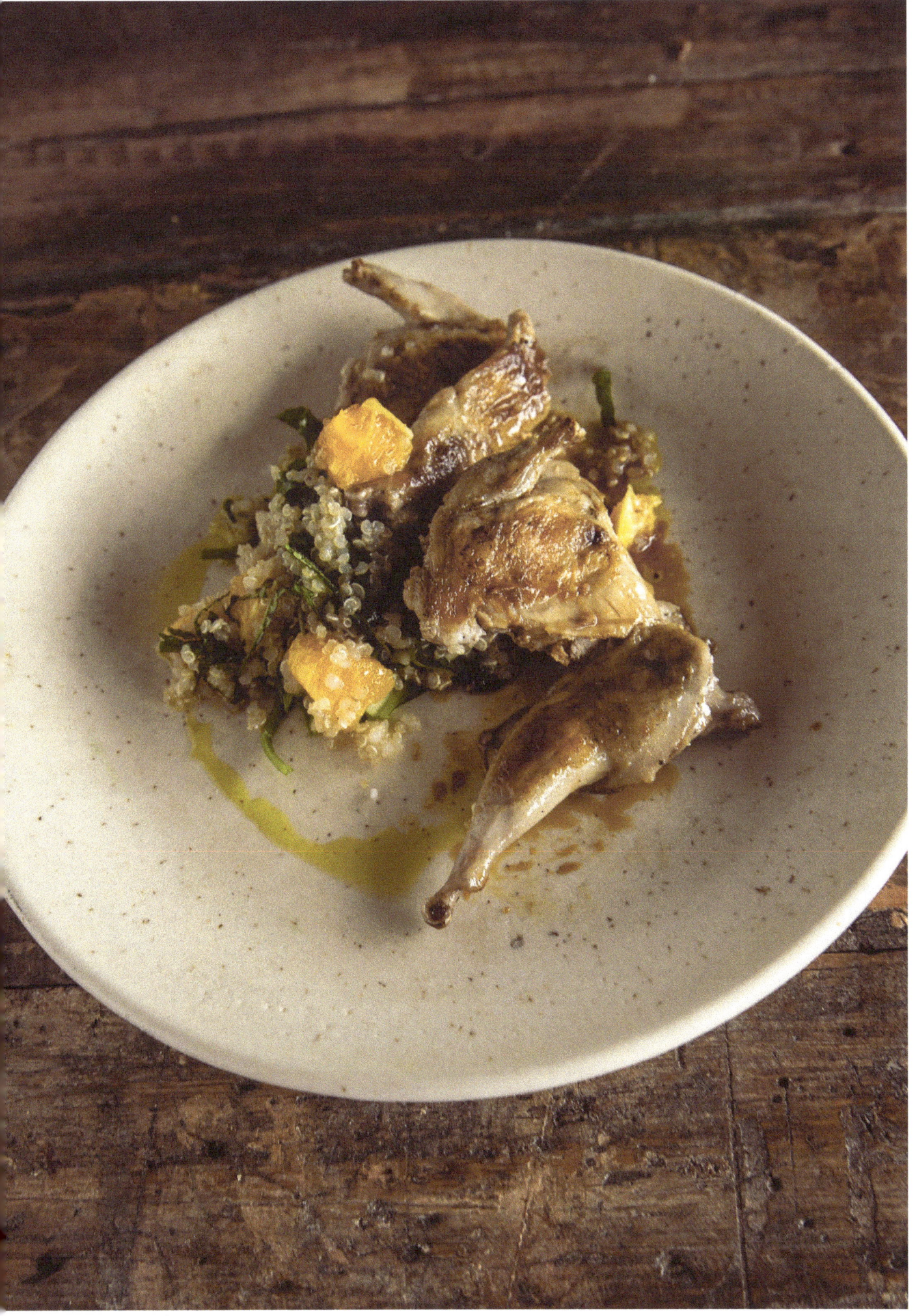

Tassal Hot Smoked Salmon, Blue Cheese, Rocket and Apple Salad with a Honey and Mustard Dressing

SERVES 2

Hot smoked salmon freezes well and is an excellent choice for a quick weeknight meal or a no-fuss impressive dinner party dish. I have chosen a delicate olive oil for the dressing of this salad to compliment the honey and creamy blue cheese.

DRESSING

1 tablespoon delicate extra virgin olive oil

½ teaspoon dijon mustard

½ teaspoon honey

1 teaspoon white wine vinegar

sea salt

white pepper

SALAD

2 red apples

2 cups rocket leaves

80 grams mild and creamy blue cheese such as King Island Roaring Forties Blue

150 gram packet Tassal Hot Smoked Salmon

To make the dressing, mix the oil, dijon mustard, honey and vinegar together well and season with salt and pepper.

To make the salad, cut the apple from the core and slice into 2mm thick batons. Wash and drain the rocket leaves. Mix the rocket leaves, apple, crumbled blue cheese and broken up salmon pieces together in a large bowl.

Just before serving, toss through the salad dressing and serve.

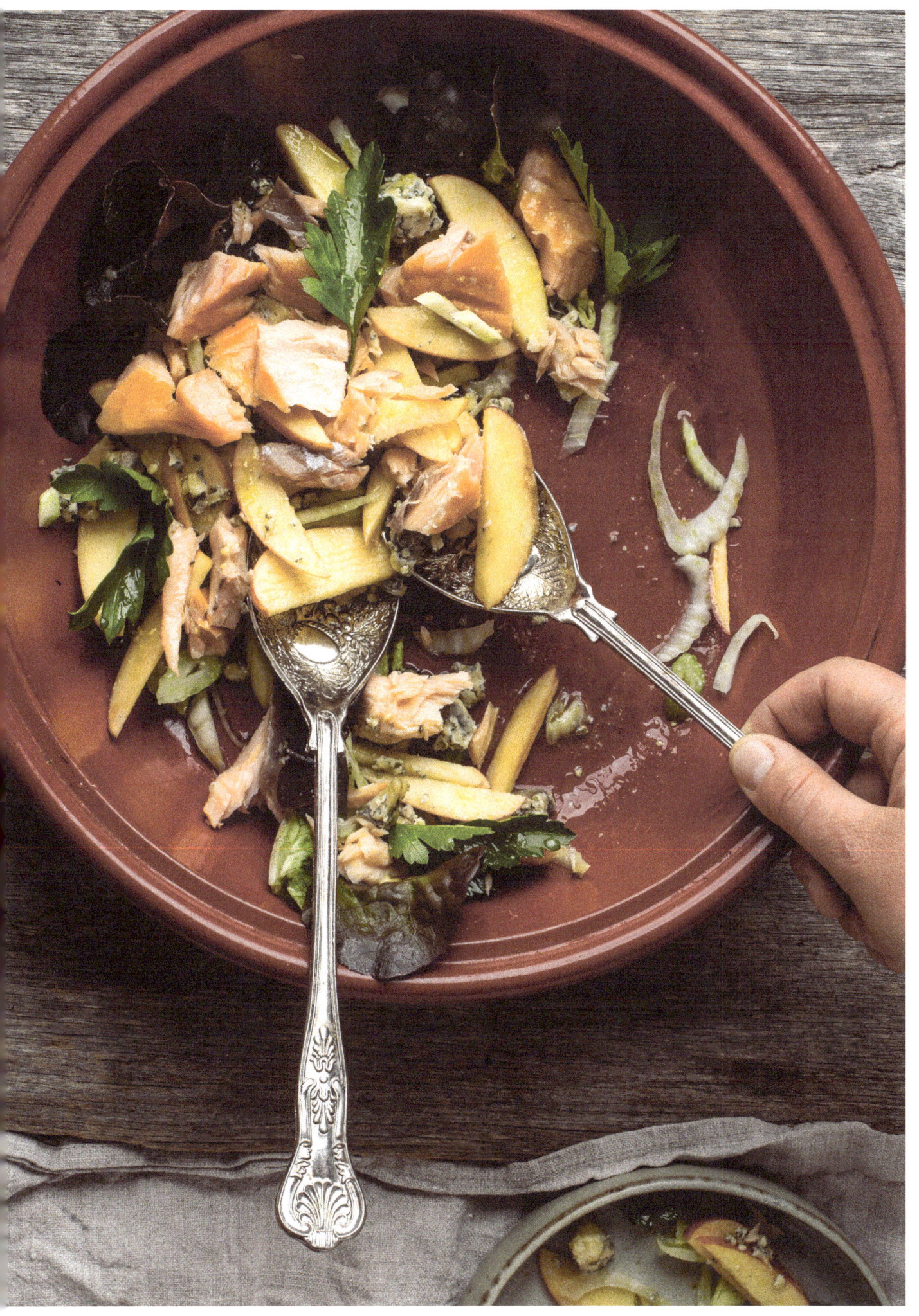

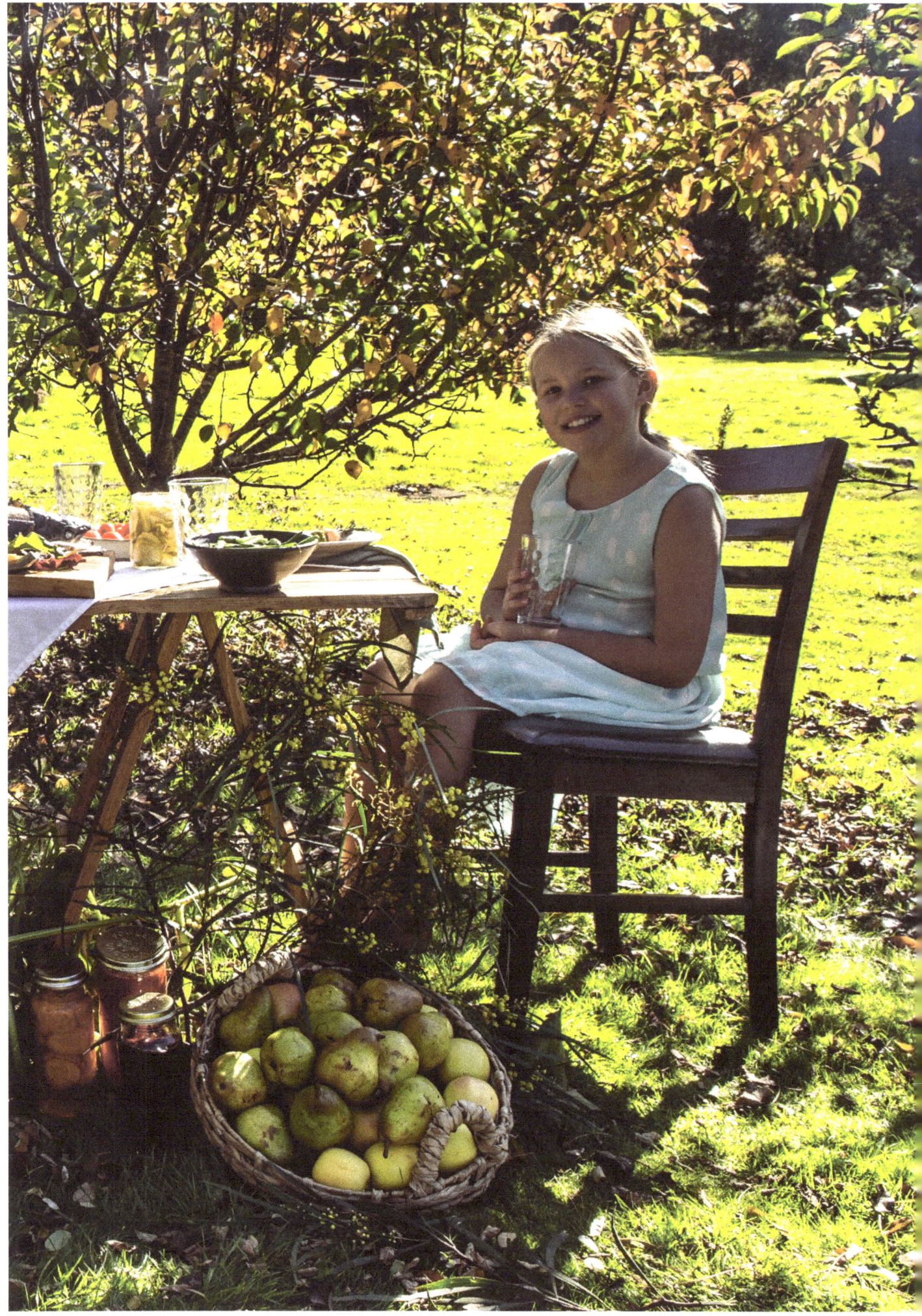

"My Nan always said a daily dose crisp fresh air was essential for a child's development. When my children were babies I would rug them up and place them in a bouncer on the deck, even during cold Tasmanian winters. Now they're older, outdoor dining is always a good opportunity for that daily dose of fresh air."

Frozen Van Diemans Land Creamery Salted Caramel Tiramisu

SERVES 12

This is a beautiful summer dessert made with Tasmania's best ice cream. This recipe uses Van Diemans Land Creamery salted caramel which is my daughter Stephanie's all time favourite ice cream. With the preparation done the day before it will make a simple and impressive dessert. We are using the lady finger biscuits for simplicity but you can make or use a simple sponge.

100ml Kahlua (optional)

100ml Amaretto (optional)

800ml Van Diemans Land Creamery vanilla ice cream

1 packet lady finger biscuits (or make a sponge)

6 shots coffee or 100ml strong coffee

800ml Van Diemans Land Creamery salted caramel ice cream

200 grams grated chocolate

Find a suitable container that is freezer safe, that will hold about 2 kilograms and when the tiramisu is turned out, you can slice it evenly. A long deep rectangle dish or container will work well.

Line the container with baking paper or cling film. If using Kahlua and Amaretto, mix the Amaretto into the vanilla ice cream and put the Kahlua in with the coffee. Spread half of the vanilla ice cream on the bottom of your freezer proof container to make the first layer.

Using around half the biscuits for the next layer, dip each biscuit in the coffee but not for too long so they are wet but not soggy and lay them on the vanilla ice cream. On top of the biscuits spread a layer of salted caramel ice cream and another layer of the soaked biscuits.

Put the last layer of vanilla ice cream on top and sprinkle with the grated chocolate. Cover the dish and freeze at least overnight.

Turn the frozen tiramisu out to serve and slice.

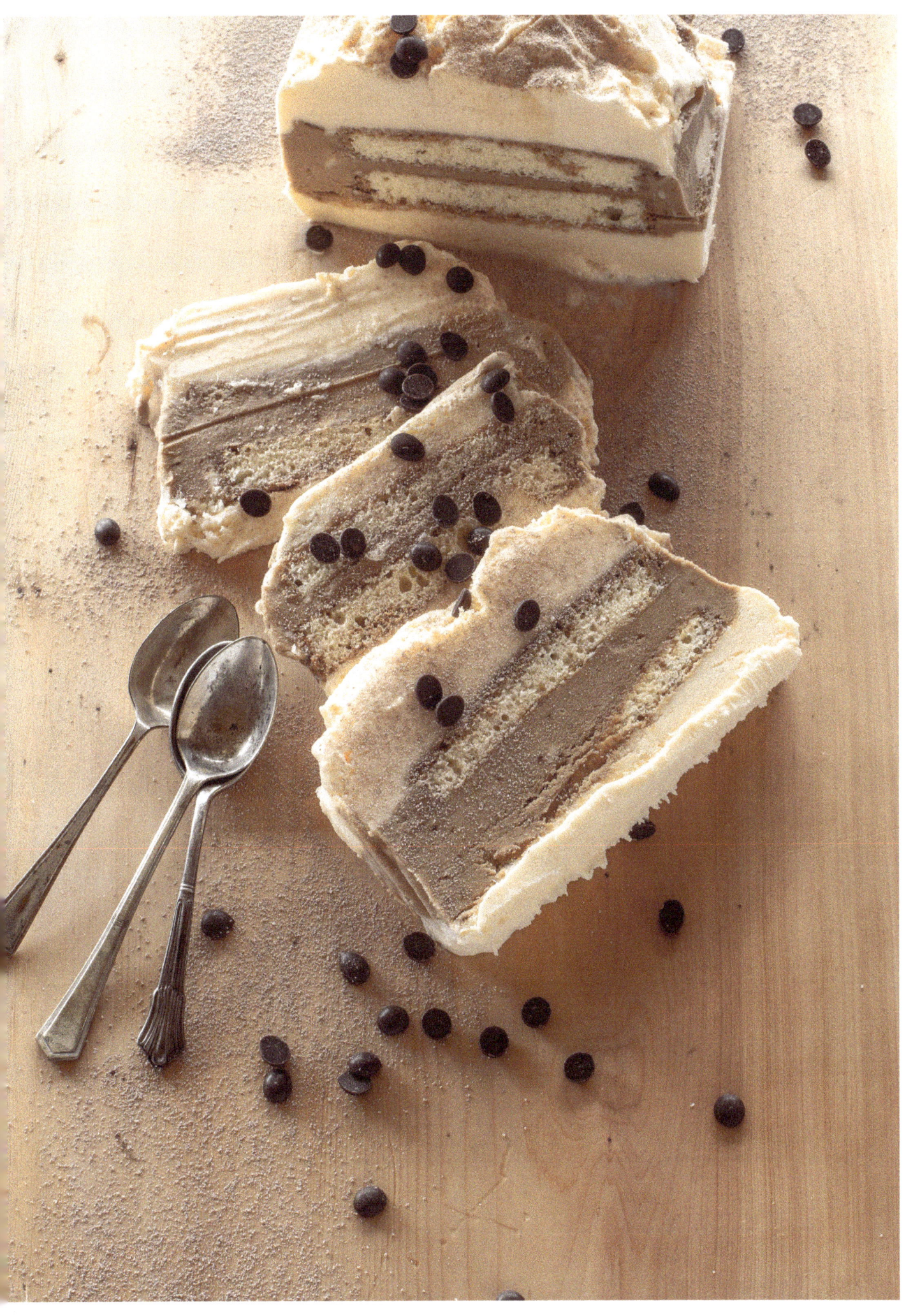

Summerlea Farm Flat Iron Steak Marinated in Preserved Lemon, Green Pepper and Horseradish

SERVES 4

This simple marinade is perfect for this gorgeous cut of meat so you can really enjoy the flavour of the steak. Serve with fat chips and Zucchini and Tomato Stew (See next page).

3 tablespoons green peppercorns

1 tablespoon preserved lemon skin

1 tablespoon horseradish

1 tablespoon thyme

1 tablespoon rosemary

1 tablespoon sage

2 tablespoons parsley

3 tablespoons robust extra virgin olive oil

600-800 grams flat iron steak

Try to get your marinade on the steak at least 24 hours before you want to cook it, this can be done up to 3 days before. To make the marinade, wash and then roughly crush the peppercorns, finely dice the preserved lemon, grate the horseradish, roughly chop the herbs and mix all together with the olive oil. Coat the steak well with the marinade and put it in a sealable container in the fridge, turning or mixing every few hours to give the steak an even coating of marinade.

To cook the steak, heat a barbeque, grill or pan to a high heat and seal the steak on each side (a few minutes) until brown and caramelised. Lower the heat to continue cooking the steak until it reaches your desired doneness. Alternatively, after browning the steak, place the steak on a tray in a preheated oven – 180C for 12 minutes for medium rare. The best method to check is with a meat thermometer - the internal temperature should be 63C for medium rare. Do resist the temptation to repeatedly poke the steak as moisture will be lost with every jab. Wrap the steak in foil to rest for at least 15 minutes before slicing and serving.

FAT CHIPS

500 grams roasting or chip potatoes (pink eye, nicola)

extra virgin olive oil

sea salt

Wash the potatoes - I pretty much never peel vegetables when I can get away with it - cut the potatoes in half if they are small or 1-2cm chunky slices. Put the potatoes in a large sauce pan and just cover with water bring to the boil on the stove and simmer for a few minutes until the potatoes are just tender when poking with a skewer. Drain.

Heat a pan on a low to medium heat, or the flat grill of the barbeque will work well, and heat then extra virgin olive oil, cook the potatoes until crisp on each side and completely cooked through and soft on the insides, around 10 minutes each side. Sprinkle with sea salt to serve.

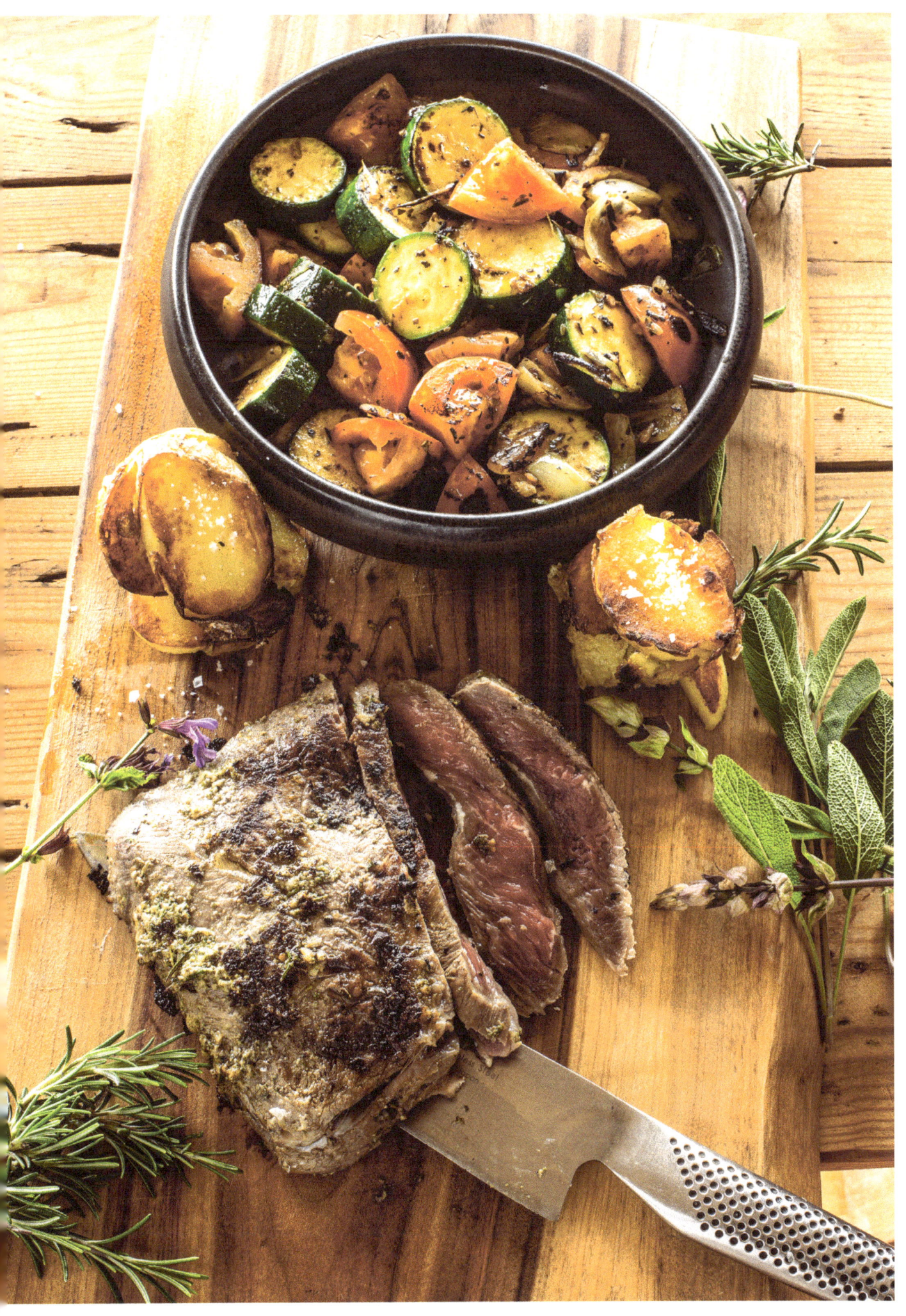

Zucchini and Tomato Stew

SERVES 4

No matter how crappy a year you have had in the garden, there will mostly always be an abundance of zucchini. If not, your neighbours and friends will be trying to give them away or they are affordable at the market for a long time. I love this simplified Ratatouille made with ingredients we grow well in Tasmania. You could also serve this as a vegetarian dish with some lentils or beans added, or throw through some pasta or serve with chicken or fish.

1 brown onion

1 tablespoon robust extra virgin olive oil

2 large zucchinis

3 cloves garlic

1 tablespoon basil

1 tablespoon oregano

sea salt

pepper

4 large tomatoes

Peel and dice the onion and peel and crush the garlic and saute them in a large heavy based pan with the olive oil for a few minutes until soft.

Add the zucchini that has been sliced into 5mm pieces and the tomato that has been roughly chopped into 1cm pieces to the pot with the herbs and salt and pepper.

Cook for about 20 minutes until the zucchini and tomato is cooked.

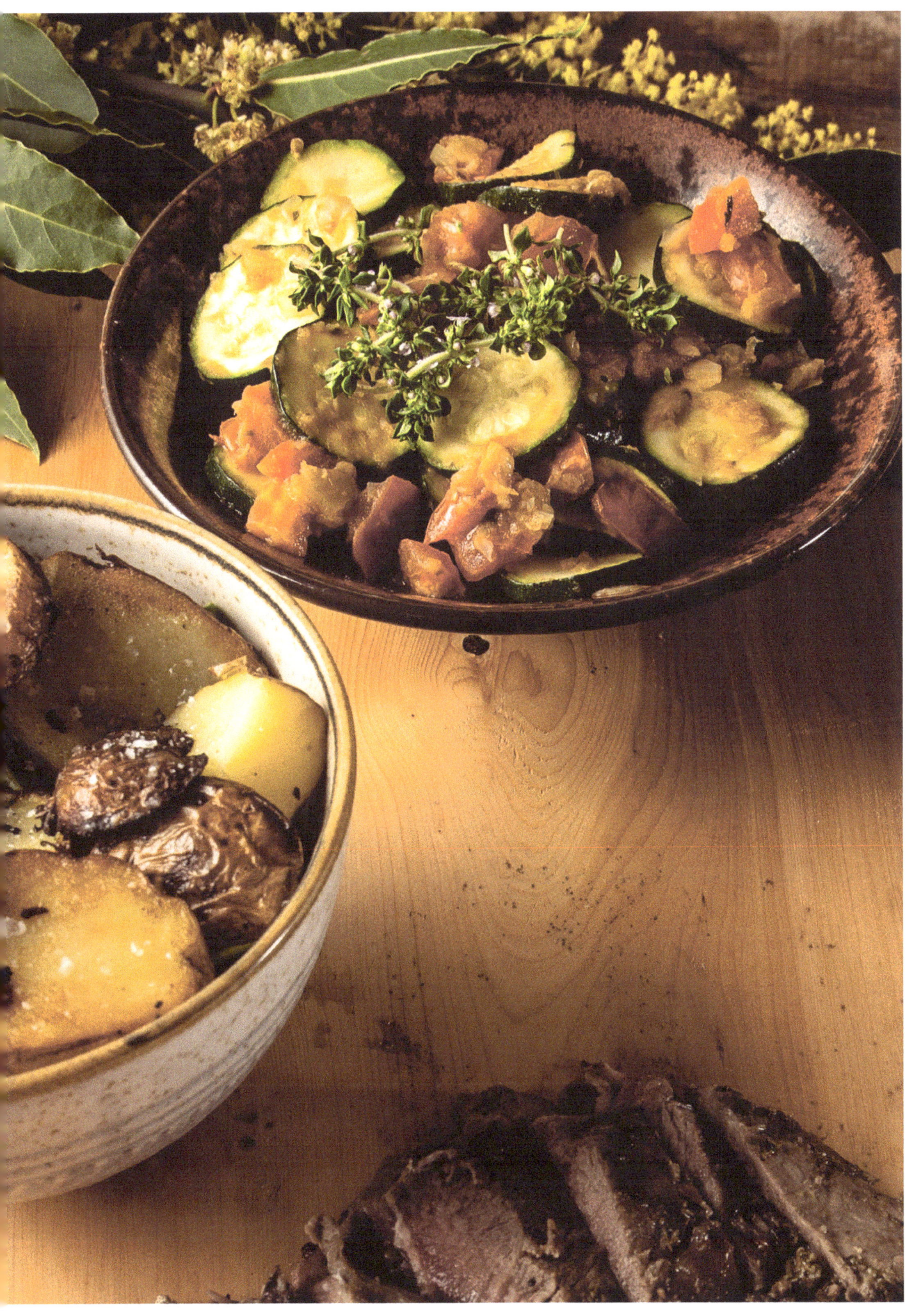

Campo De Flori Lavender Aioli with Crayfish Bruschetta

SERVES 4-6

When cooking with lavender you can use the extracted oil or the dried flowers. For a recipe like this one when we want a subtle flavour the dried flowers works best. The flowers have a subtle flavour that increase the intensity the longer it is steeped in a liquid solution. With the delicate soft flavours of crayfish, we want the accompanying aioli to have a hint of the beautiful lavender and not be over powering, so add the lavender and make the aioli close to serving (within the hour). Use a delicate or medium extra virgin olive oil such as Wattle Hill Boutillon. This stunning aioli can be served with many different dishes such as crispy fried chicken, crumbed and fried fish fillets, vegetable fritters, cooked cheeses or spiced cauliflower.

1 cooked crayfish

4 x 1cm thick slices sourdough

2 apples

1 large kohlrabi

½ bunch Italian parsley

1 tablespoon cider vinegar

1 tablespoon delicate extra virgin olive oil

sea salt

white pepper

AIOLI

1 teaspoon dried Campo De Flori Lavender

1 egg yolk

pinch sea salt

pinch white pepper

1 tablespoon apple cider vinegar

100ml delicate extra virgin olive oil (approximately)

Toast or grill the sourdough slices brushed with a little extra virgin olive oil. Slice the apples and kohlrabi into slices and then into thin sticks, roughly chop the parsley. Mix the apple, kohlrabi, parsley with the vinegar and oil and season with the salt and pepper. Assemble the dressed salad onto each piece of sourdough, top with the sliced crayfish meat and drizzle with the aioli.

To make the aioli, in the thermocooker or a blender or with a bowl whisk and strong fast-moving arm, add the yolk, vinegar and lavender and blitz, now pour the oil in a slow thin stream while continually blending or whisking to create a thick sauce.

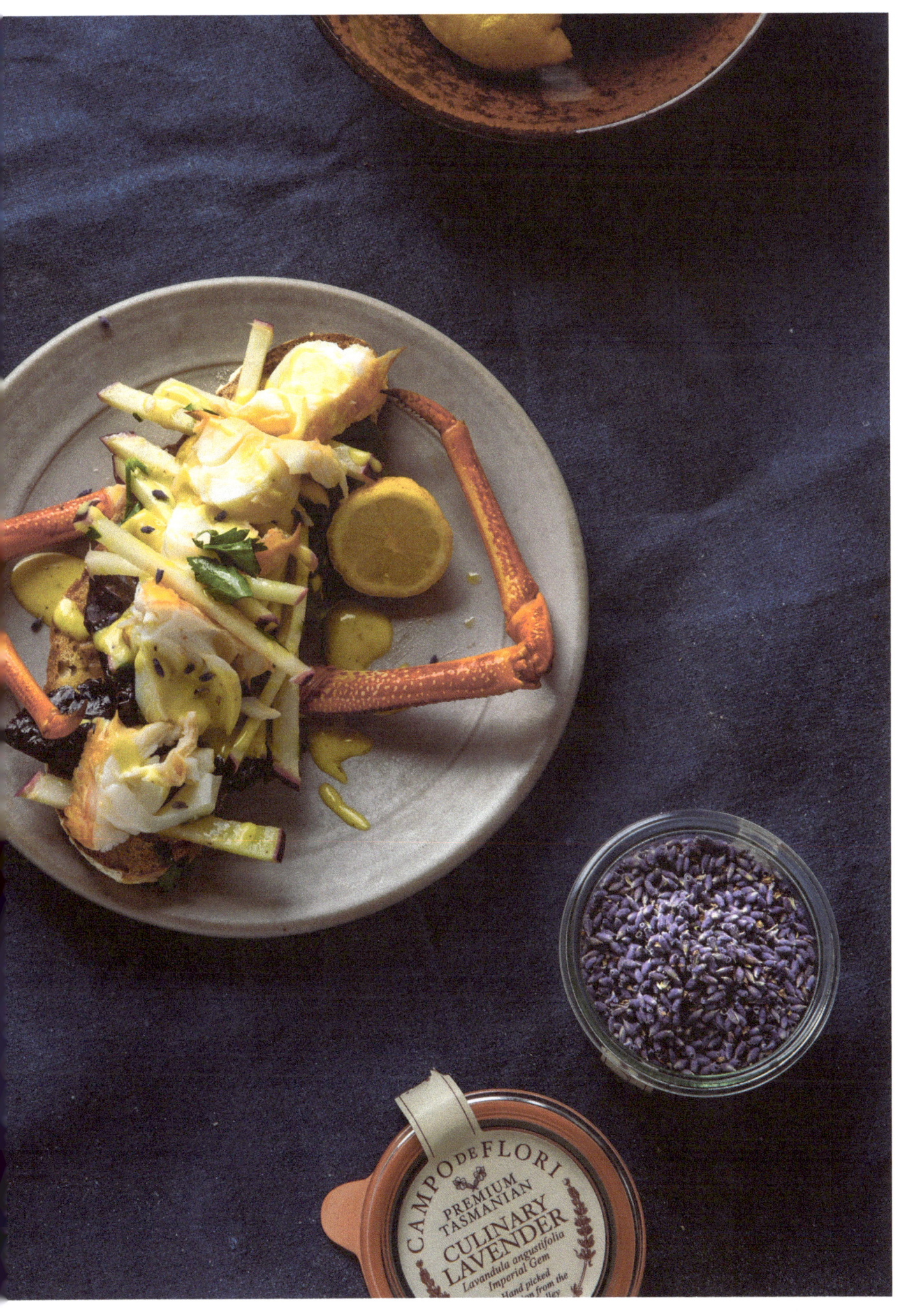

Raw Striped Trumpeter Kohlrabi Quick Pickle

SERVES 4

This white fleshed fish is best served raw when fresh. It's always exciting for us to get the first stripy for the season at the start of summer. Brendan knows the first few are for us and not to be sold, no matter how desperate the bank account is looking! Kohlrabi is a beautiful vegetable that is part of the brassica family I find I use it similarly to a radish or cabbage, it is beautiful in a slaw, sautéed with olive oil or in salads. This quick pickle adds heaps of flavour but does not lose the crunch and flavour of the veggie. This recipe is the perfect example of when simplicity is best, and what an easy but impressive dish to create for a dinner party.

200 grams fresh striped trumpeter fillet no skins or bones

1 kohlrabi

50ml rice wine vinegar

50 grams sugar

1 tablespoon lemon

extra virgin olive oil to serve

To make the quick pickle simply heat the rice wine vinegar and dissolve the sugar, peel and finely slice the kohlrabi. Once the syrup is cooled put the kohlrabi in and leave for a few hours.

To prepare the fish simply slice and serve with the kohlrabi and a drizzle of extra virgin olive oil.

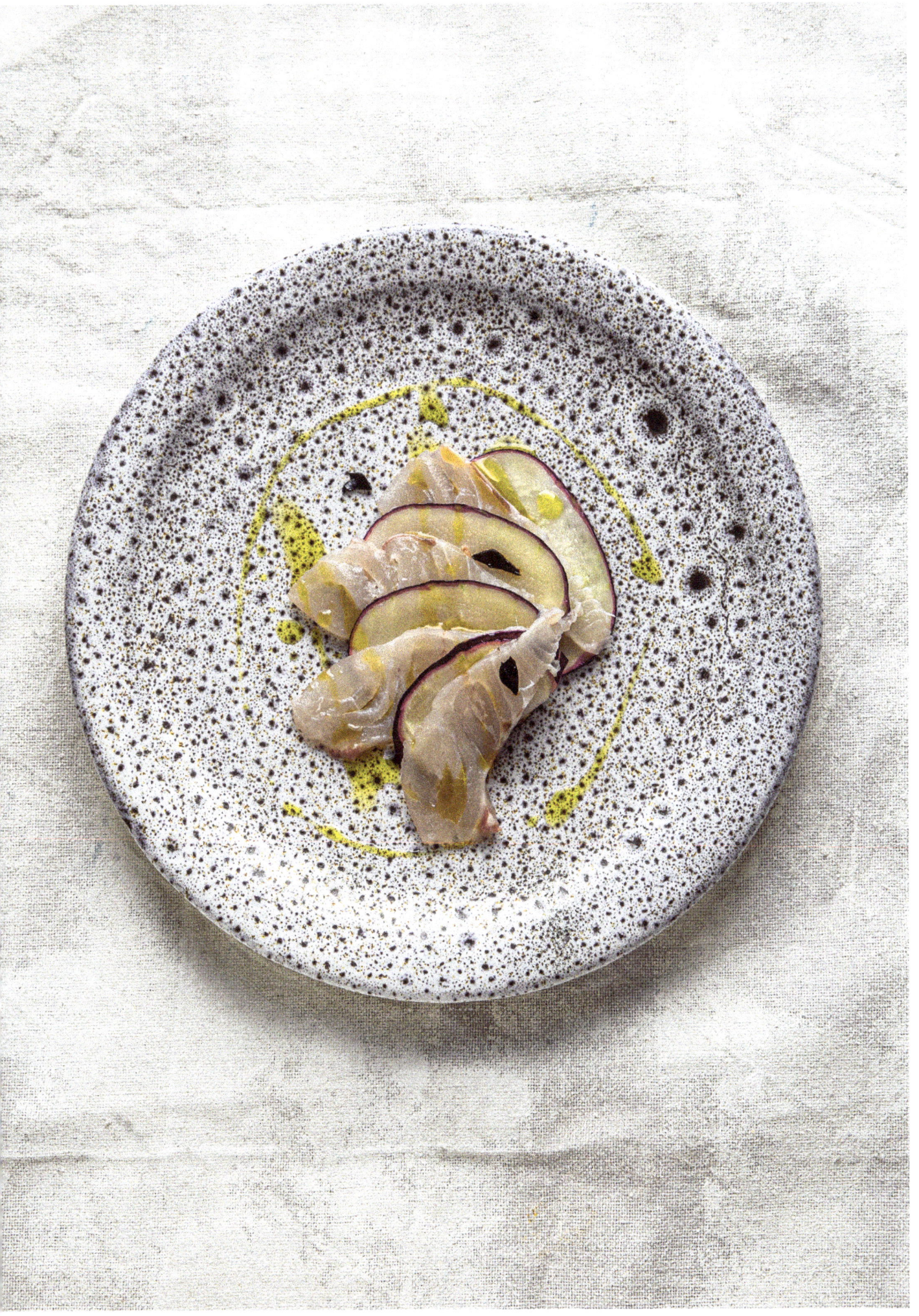

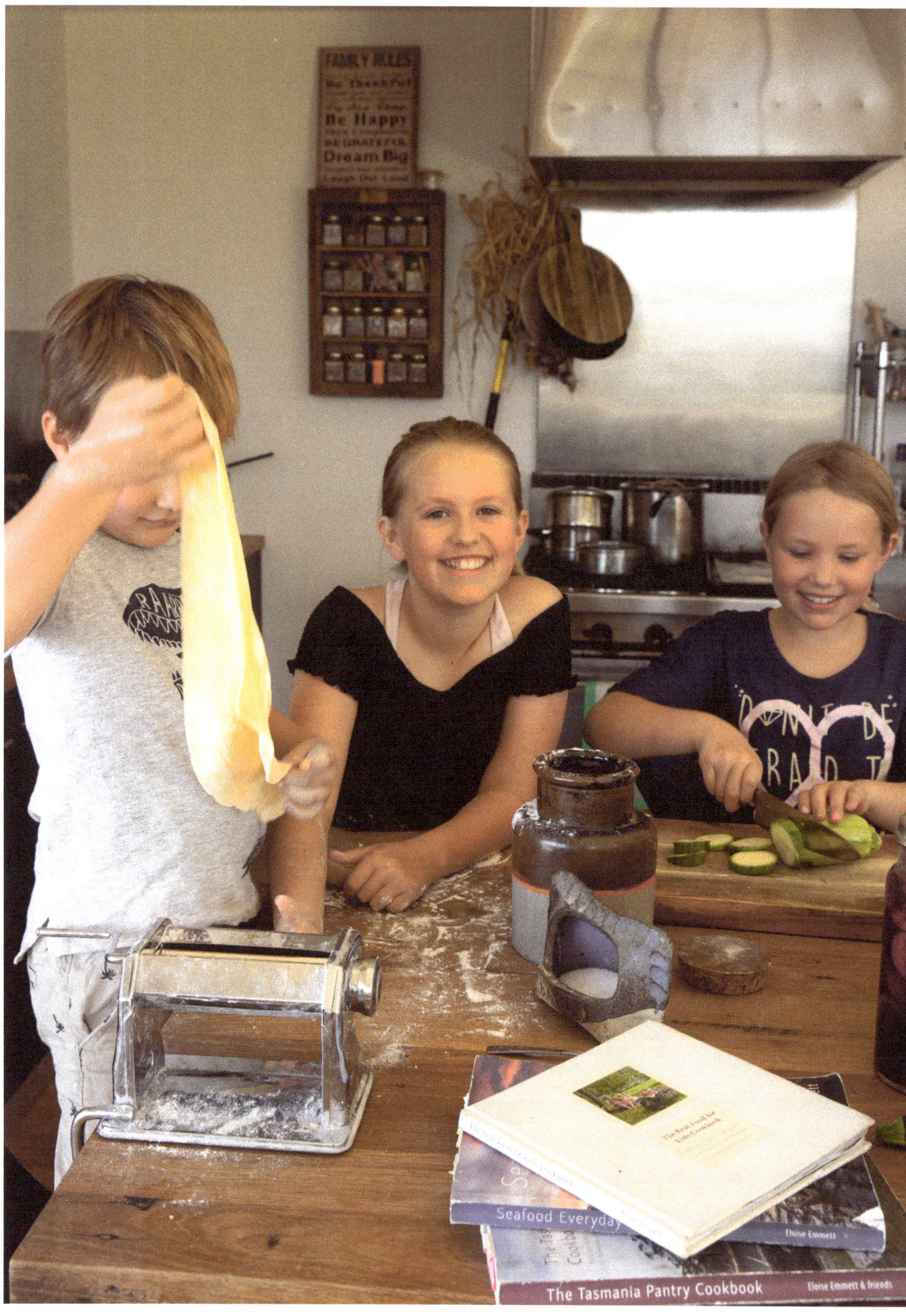

"Big food companies have convinced us that cooking is hard, so we buy their packaged plastic food full of cheap and nasty ingredients."

Striped Trumpeter Confit

SERVES 4

If you are going to cook this beautiful white fleshed fish then I think this is the absolute best method. I choose a delicate extra virgin olive oil for this dish as we don't want the olive oil to be over powering. Wattle Hill Boutillon is one of the most delicate in flavour olive oils I have found in Tasmania. I don't want to waste a drop of the oil so after cooking, the oil is used to dress the salad. It is wise to squeeze the fish in the smallest pan that you can fit them in, so that it does not take too much oil to cover the fillets. If you did have oil left over after cooking, then simply strain it, pop it in a jar and refrigerate it and use it again to cook with other seafood. Extra virgin olive oil can handle 6 hours of cooking before it loses any of its incredible health benefits, so at my home the leftover oil would be used to fry some crumbed fish and pinkeye potato chips in the following few days.

4 x 200 gram striped trumpeter portions

delicate extra virgin olive oil

2 medium carrots

1 kohlrabi

1 fennel bulb

6 brocoletti

20 snow peas

½ bunch parsley

1 lemon

sea salt

white pepper

To cook the fish, find the smallest heavy base pan you can squeeze the fish into and brush the base with the oil. Squeeze in the fish and just cover with the olive oil. Put on the stove top to the lowest possible temperature, even move the pan slightly to the side to get a lower temperature. Oil should be at below 90°C for about 30 minutes until the fish is just set.

While the fish is cooking prepare the salad by peeling and finely slicing into skinny batons the carrot, fennel, brocoletti and de stringing the peas, and slice, shred the parsley. Toss in a bowl with the lemon juice, and season well with a good pinch of white pepper and sea salt, assemble the salad onto a serving platter and place the hot fish on top with a few scoops of the hot oil to dress the salad. Serve immediately.

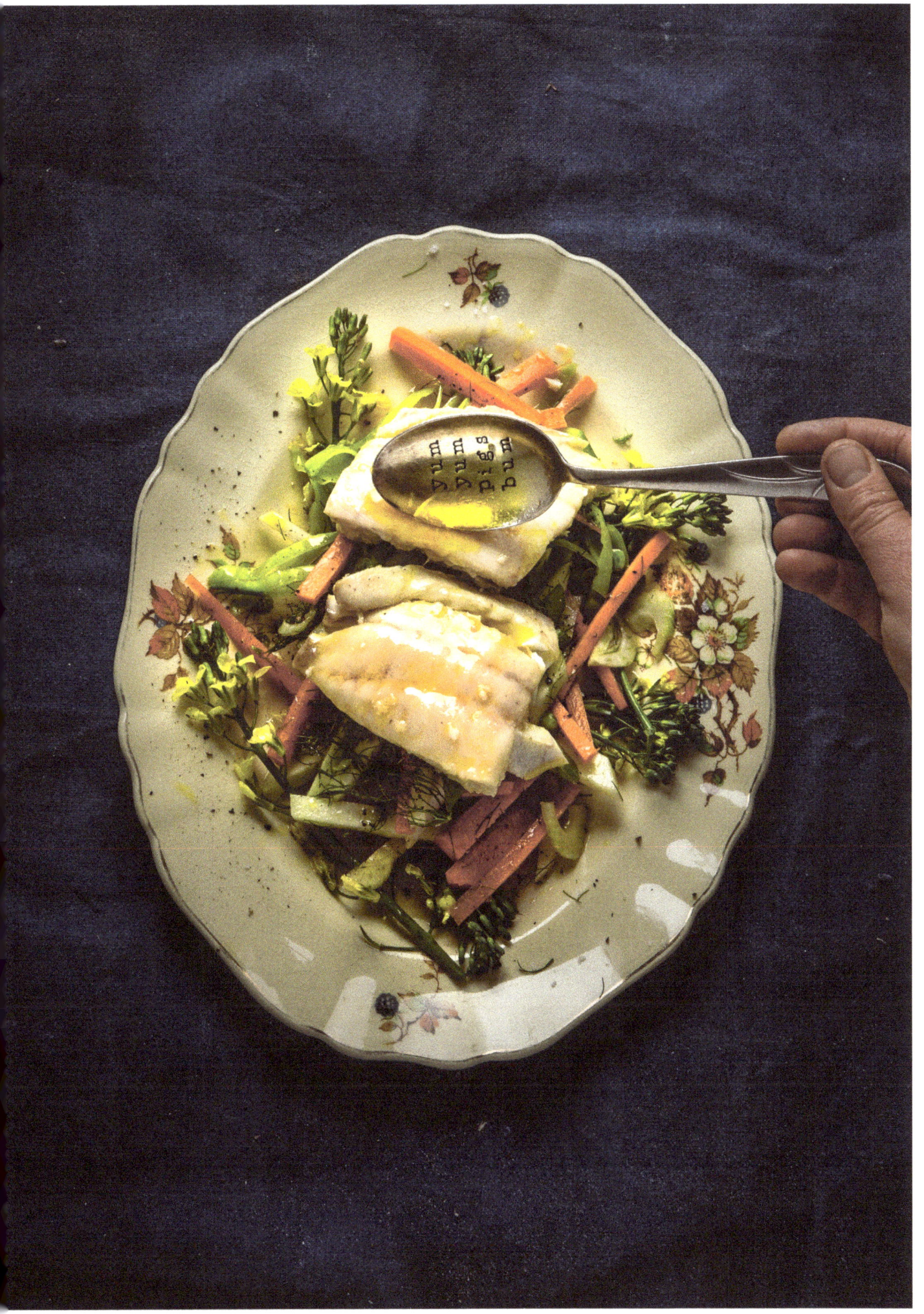

Parrot Fish Hong Kong Style

SERVES 4

Wrasse or parrot fish is one of the fish my husband Brendan catches commercially. The fish are keep alive after he catch's them and they are held in aerated tanks and flown to Melbourne and Sydney to swim around in tanks in Chinese restaurants. I never really knew what the fuss was about and was always a bit baffled by why they were worth so much on the restaurant menus on visits to Melbourne and Sydney. In a cooking demonstration, I was delighted to hear Tetsuya say parrot fish was his favourite fish and even more excited to see him cook one at the 2019 Australian Wooden Boat Festival Tasmanian Seafood Industry Council Kitchen Theatre. This is an adaption of his recipe and method. I have since researched it and it is a popular method for lots of different seafood. I have tried this recipe with other whole fresh fish and salmon fillets, oysters and half shell scallops, and they were all delicious.

1 wrasse, head on, gutted and scaled

6 large spring onions

2cm piece ginger

1 clove garlic

1 teaspoon fish sauce

2 tablespoons soy sauce

100ml sesame oil

A smaller fish will fit in the varoma of the thermocooker, otherwise you'll need a fish steamer or similar steaming system that will fit a large fish. A baking tray with a cake rack and lid or kitchen foil will do if you need. I steam fish regularly so have invested in a large fish steamer.

Put the fish in the steamer and water underneath the steaming rack and steam at a low temperature until the fish is cooked (or almost) through to the bone.

While the fish is steaming finely slice the spring onion, garlic, ginger and mix with the soy and fish sauces.

Put the sesame oil in a small pan and heat until smoking.

Remove the fish from the steamer and assemble on a platter with the spring onion garnish on top and pour the smoking hot oil over the garnish and serve.

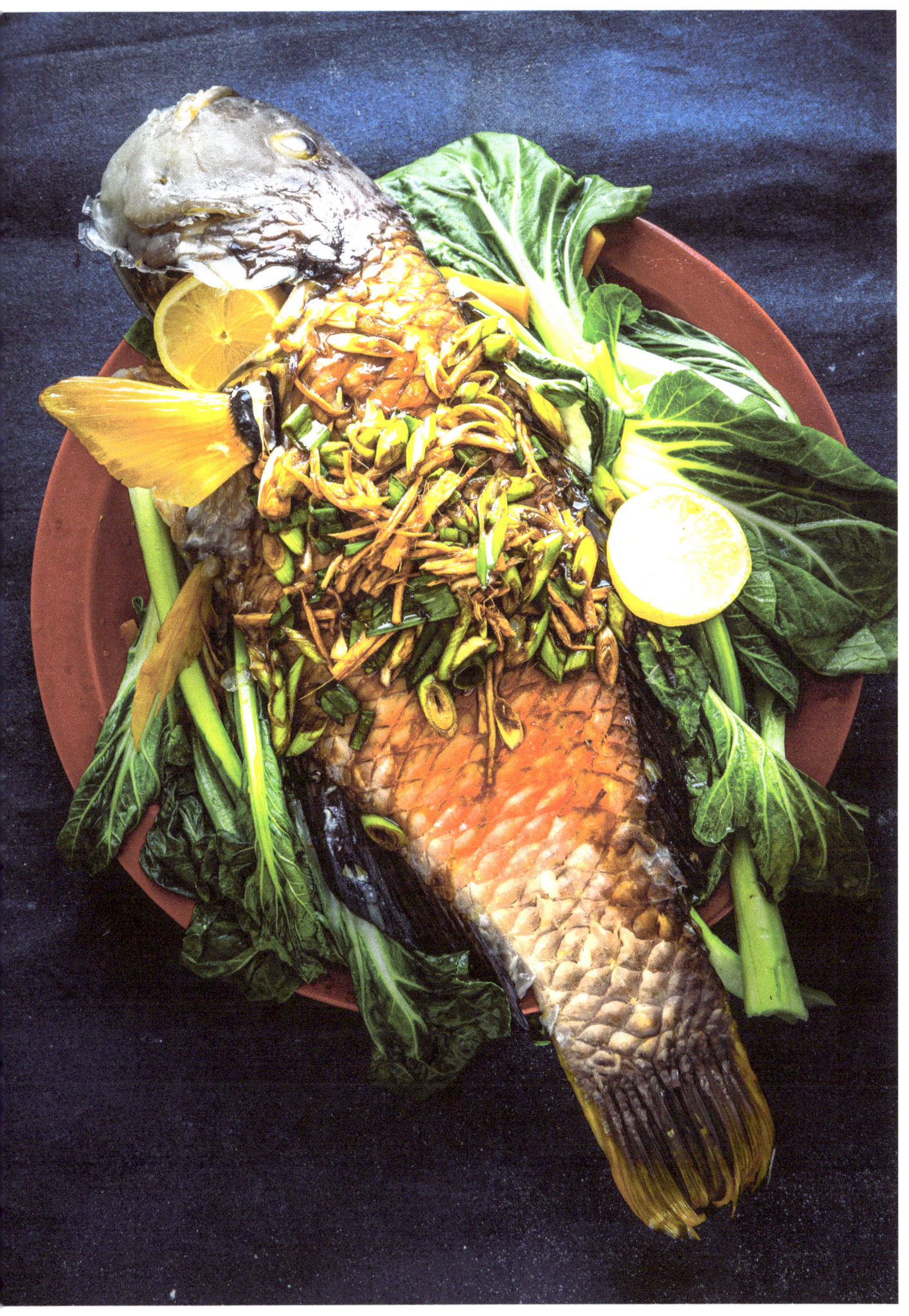

Salmon and Saffron Butter

SERVES A FEAST

Salmon and saffron is a match made in heaven. Rich and creamy saffron butter melting through salmon that is only just cooked and moist is hard to beat. Serve the whole salmon for a feast for many. The butter can be easily rolled and frozen and then slices cut off when needed, to simply grab a few slices to serve on baked or steamed salmon. This is not hard or time consuming to make, but start steeping the saffron in the cream at least a day before making the butter to achieve a more intense flavour. Serve with some smashed potato or boiled new season pinkeyes and a simple salad or some steamed greens. Order your fish from the Tassal Salmon Shop to make sure they have a whole fish in when you need it.

500ml cream

a good pinch of Campo De Flori saffron threads

sea salt

1 whole salmon, head on, gutted or fillets

To make the butter seep the saffron in the cream at least overnight. Then beat the cream with the salt until the butter has separated from the butter milk. Keep the butter milk for pikelets, scones, pancakes or bread. Roll the butter between plastic wrap and refrigerate.

If you are baking a whole salmon make sure the fish is gutted and scaled. Heat the oven to 160°C. For presentation lay the salmon on its belly and push the belly flaps out. Brush with extra virgin olive oil and season with salt and pepper and bake in the oven for around 30 minutes - this is going to depend on the size of the fish.

It is best to aim for a medium doneness as it will continue to cook. To check if to see if it is cooked to your liking, poke the top at the spine with a fork and you should be able to wiggle the fin out. When it's ready, slice the skin on top and fold back and lay the butter on top to serve, so that the butter melts through the flesh.

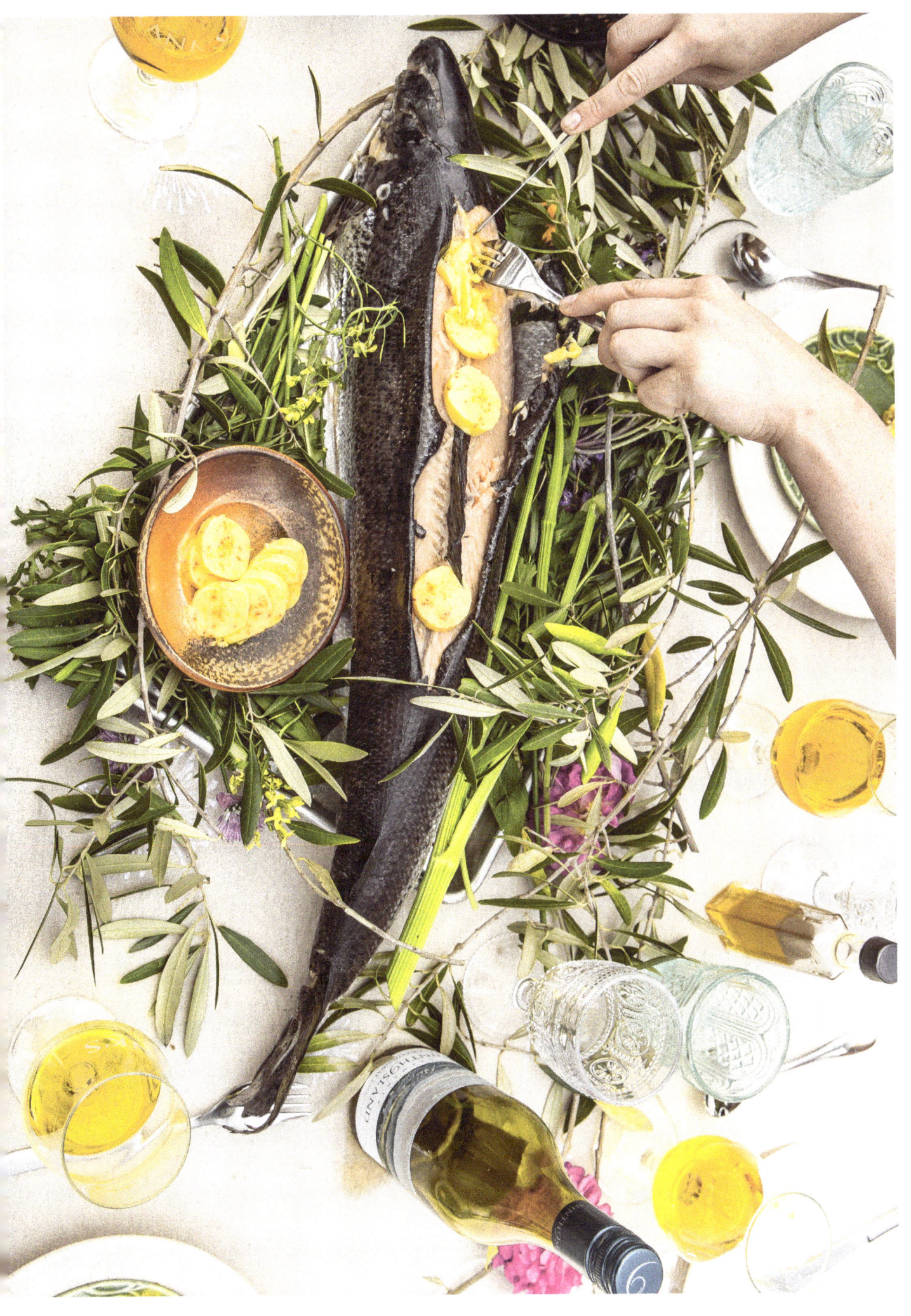

Sourdough

I am fascinated by sourdough. You simply ferment flour to make a loaf of well risen bread! It really is quite amazing! If you jump onto google you'll find yourself a million different methods and recipes on how to make sourdough. I am onto my fifth attempt in my life to keep a sourdough starter and make bread regularly, but this works for me and I have had this starter alive for over 4 years now! I make it work for me by keeping it simple. My loaves are probably not Instagram worthy, but they are delicious and the method is practical enough to keep it up regularly in the home kitchen.

My sourdough, in particular my olive loaf that I eat regularly for my breakfast toast, is pretty much the only bread I eat. However I do love some fluffy white bread on the odd occasion. I schedule my sourdough making on the days I'm doing lots of laundry, which I need some time to do each week anyway. If I have prepped my leaven the night before and I start early on a Sunday, I can prepare the dough for two loaves while I do some house work and catch up on laundry. I then leave them to rise for the day and at around 3pm I can get the oven on to cook a Sunday roast and prepare some other lunch box or weeknight meals whilst the bread is baking. Easy!

I then freeze the loaves cut in half or sliced. That way I only need to bake once a fortnight or once a month, with my starter living in the fridge in between baking. I find it works best when taken out of the fridge and fed for four days before it is needed. I start feeding the starter on a Tuesday morning before the Sunday bake. I have an organic unbleached wholemeal flour to feed my starter and I normally bake with white bakers flour.

PRE FERMENT

100 grams sourdough starter

100 grams flour

100 grams water

BREAD

500 grams flour

320ml water

1 tablespoon sea salt

THE STARTER

I recommend getting some starter from a friend who has been baking for a while, I am always happy to feed and share my starter. Perhaps ask a bakery, or even putting a call out on social media. I have had my started on the go now for 4 years, it seemed to take a good few months to really have the fermentation that it now has to rise my loaves. When I separate my starter off at my classes and weekend cooking retreats my guest can go home and start baking straight away.

If you HAVE to start your starter yourself, find an organic wholemeal flour that is reasonably fresh. Add 50 grams of flour and 50 grams of water to a jar and mix with your hands (to catch wild yeasts) every day. Leave the jar on the bench and feed it every day with the 50 grams of water and 50 grams of flour at around the same time each day. You should have some bubbles and be ready to prepare your leaven and bake in about a week.

When I am baking every few days, such as when we are on holidays, then I will feed my starter every day and it lives on the bench. If I won't be baking every day I'll store mine in the fridge and pull it out a few days before I am baking. Whilst in the fridge I pull it out every couple of weeks to feed it if I am not baking for a while.

Continued next page >

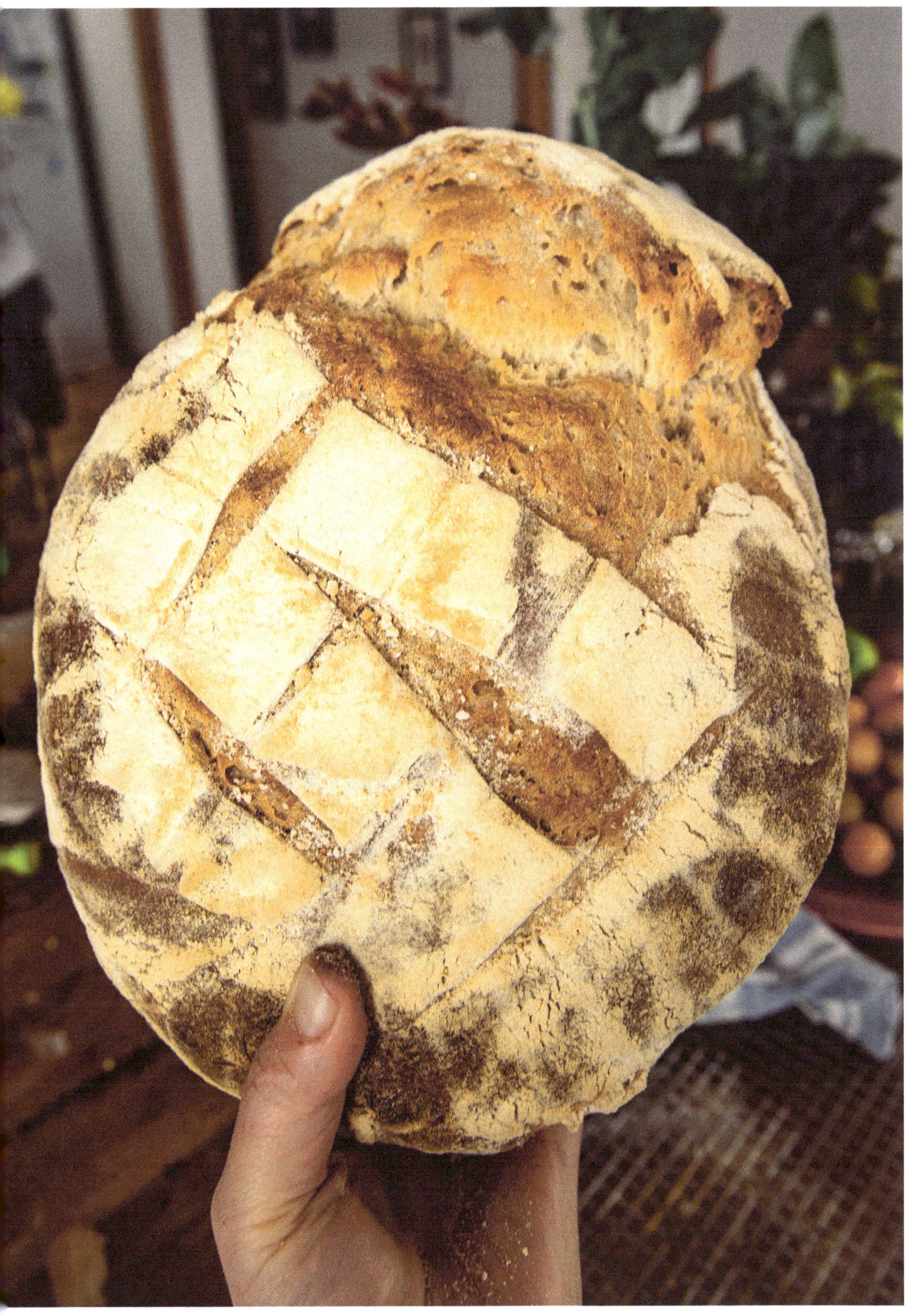

Sourdough (continued)

THE LEAVEN OR PRE-FERMENT

In the evening of the day before I am baking, I mix 100 grams starter, 100 grams flour and 100 grams water and leave overnight. I use the thermocooker for my first knead so I do this in the thermocooker bowl.

THE BREAD

Add to the preferment, 500 grams baking flour, 320ml water and a tablespoon of salt and knead well, 3 minutes in the thermocooker or mixer, or knead well by hand for about 10 minutes to form a smooth wet dough. Then do your first fold, basically pull a side out and press over the top of the dough 10 times.

Leave to rest for 25-30 minutes and do another 5 folds leaving it to rest 25-30 minutes to rest in between. Dust lightly with flour when needed. Line a colander with muslin cloth or another cloth and flour well, actually rub the flour into the cloth and put the dough in there with the seam side of the dough ball on top. Put the colander in a plastic bag to create a little warm room and leave for 4-8 hours until the dough has risen by about a third of its size, and you can see the little air bubbles.

Heat the oven as hot as you can, about 220°C. Carefully flip the dough out onto a tray and slice the top of the dough, not too deep, to prevent the crust from splitting during baking. Add a splash of water to the tray and bake for 20 minutes. Turn the oven down to 200°C and continue to bake for another 20 minutes.

Now try to leave it to cool completely before slicing, as this will keep the moisture in... impossible!! I normally cut the end off while it is still burning my fingers to create a little cup which I fill with extra virgin olive oil and a sprinkle of sea salt!

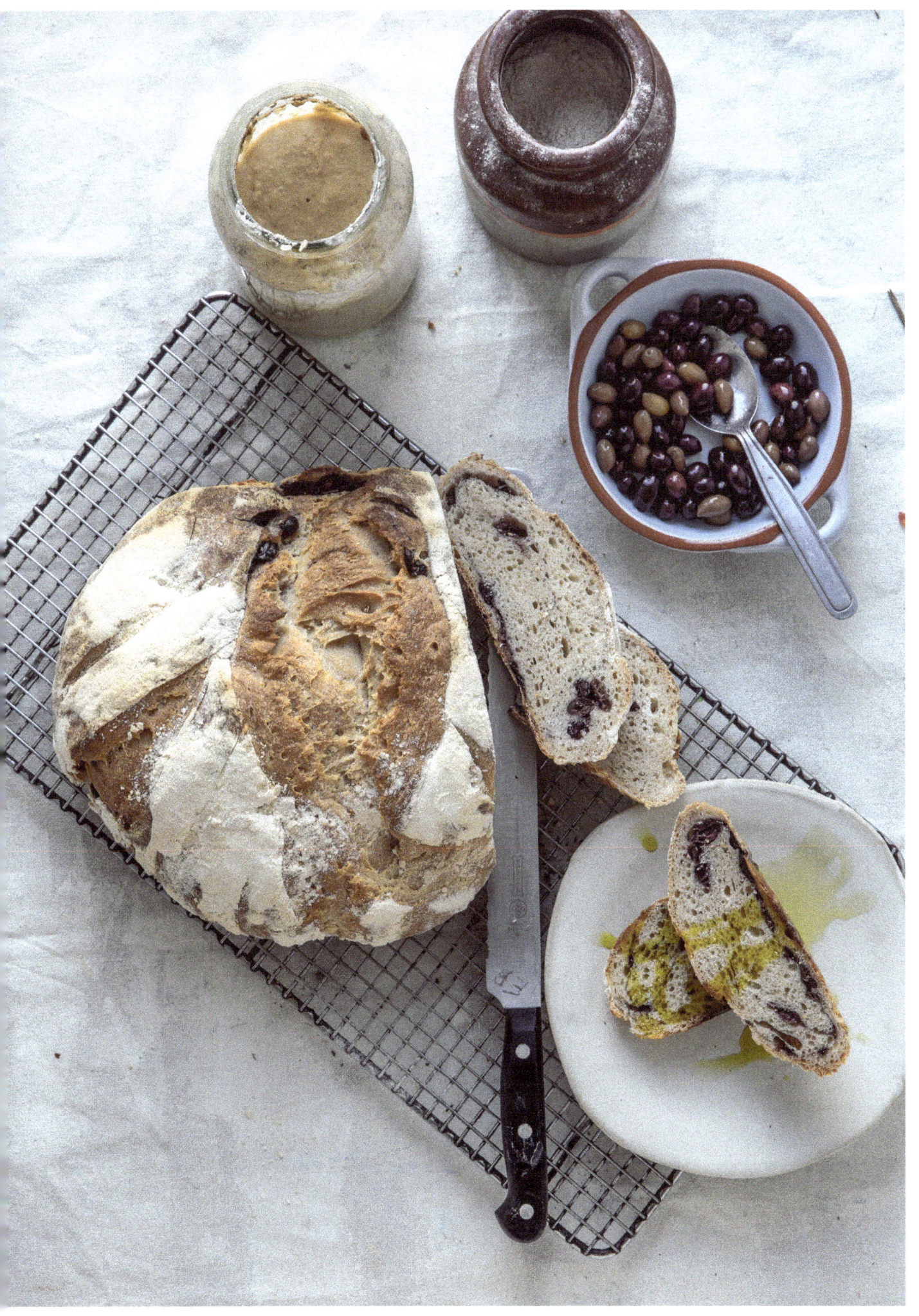

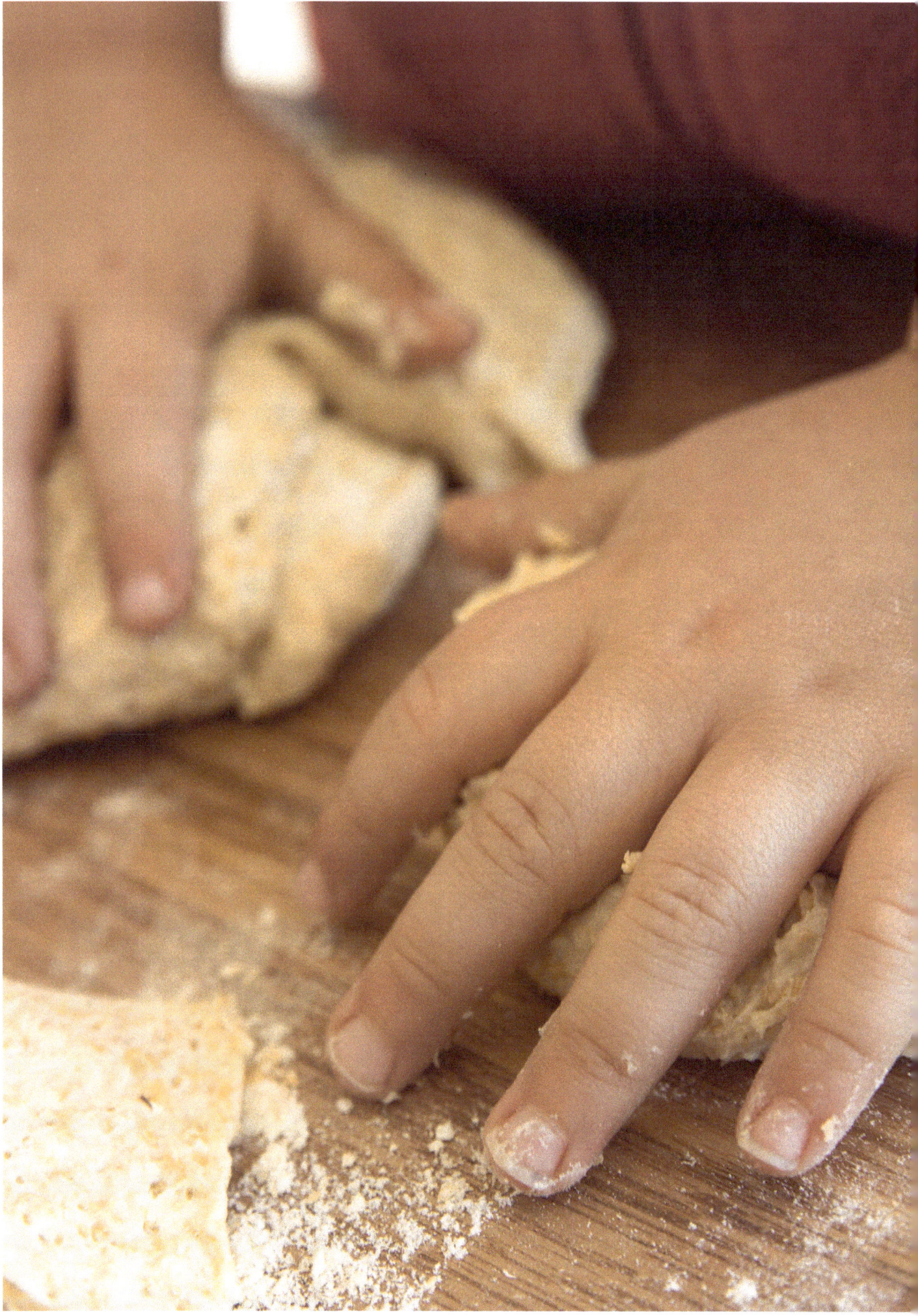

Sourdough Toast Ideas

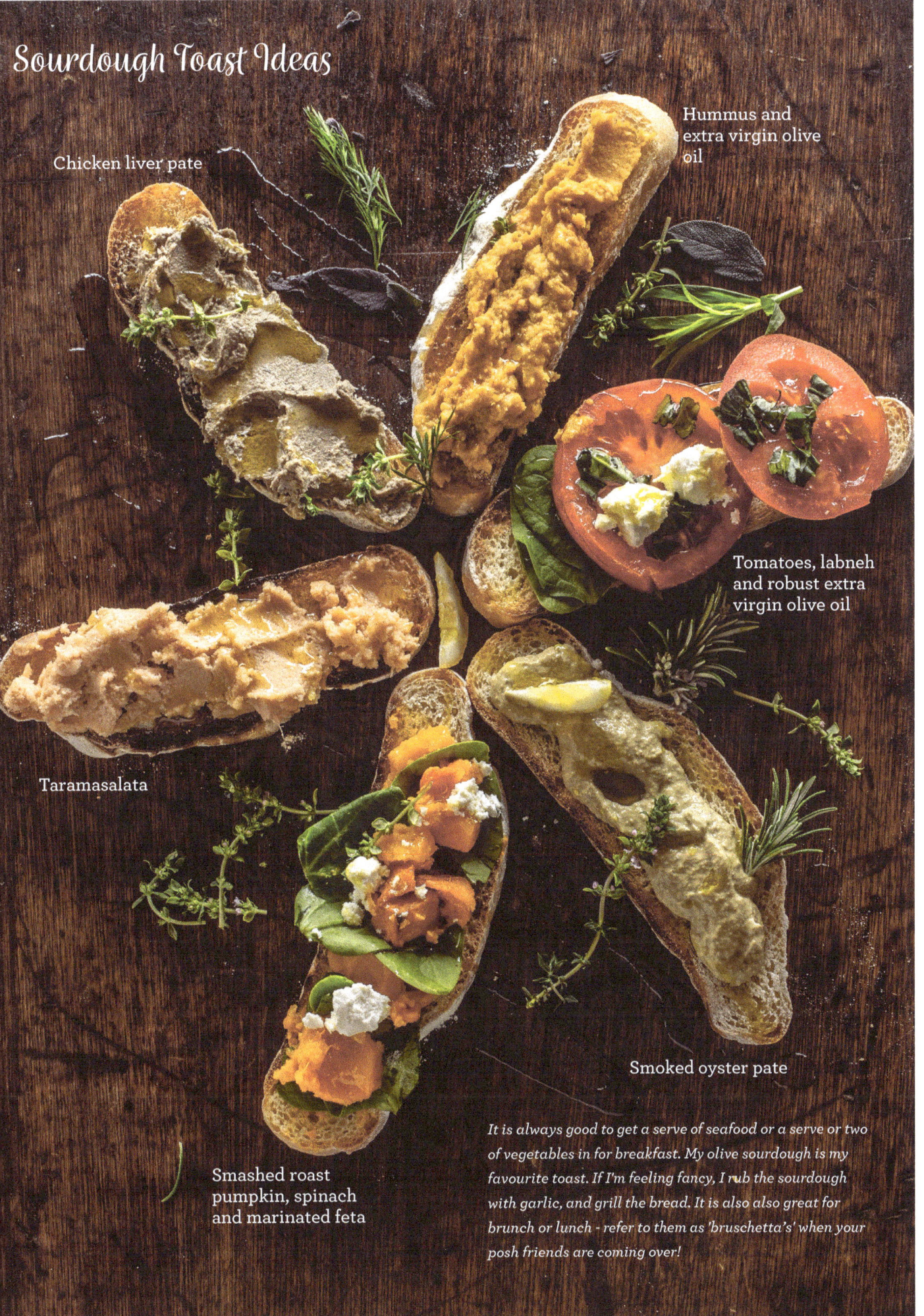

Chicken liver pate

Hummus and extra virgin olive oil

Tomatoes, labneh and robust extra virgin olive oil

Taramasalata

Smoked oyster pate

Smashed roast pumpkin, spinach and marinated feta

It is always good to get a serve of seafood or a serve or two of vegetables in for breakfast. My olive sourdough is my favourite toast. If I'm feeling fancy, I rub the sourdough with garlic, and grill the bread. It is also also great for brunch or lunch - refer to them as 'bruschetta's' when your posh friends are coming over!

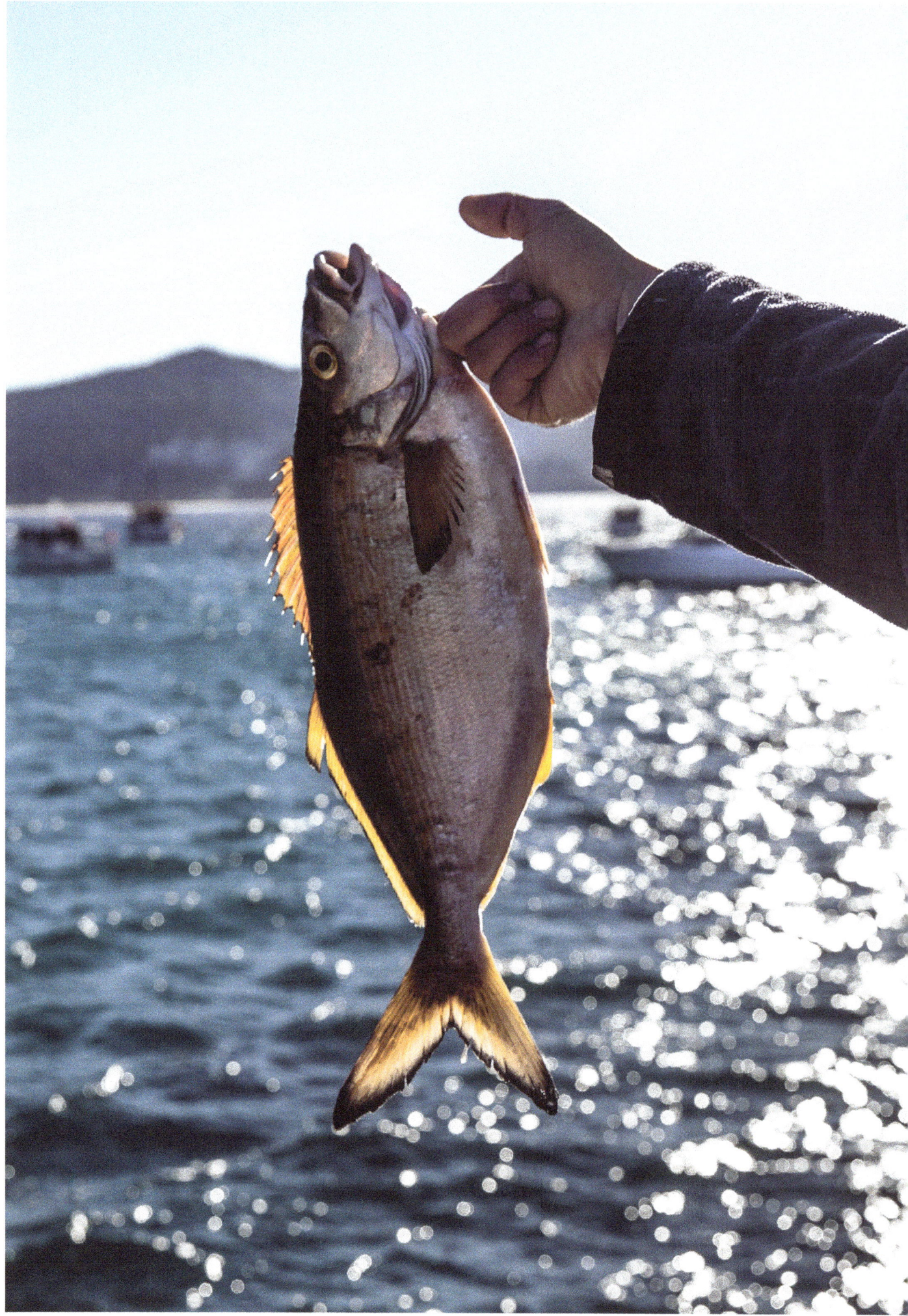

"I like to explore using different varieties of local fish. The more we support the local fish industry, it allows our produce to stay in our state."

Croissants

MAKES 12

A labour of love but absolutely essential for the special occasion breakfast! Serve simply with your home-made jams or scrambled eggs smoked salmon and brie, divine.

500 grams bakers flour

1 teaspoon salt

1 teaspoon sugar

1 teaspoon yeast

300ml - 320ml water

250 grams butter

I have written the steps out so you can move a counter (coin or piece of blue tac) and mark the recipe so you know where you are up to.

Step 1. Starting the day before you want to bake your croissants.
Make a dough exactly like a bread dough with the flour, salt, sugar yeast and lukewarm water. Knead 3 minutes in the thermocooker or mixer, or knead well by hand for about 10 minutes to form a smooth dough.

Leave in a bowl covered with plastic film to rise in a warm spot for a few hours until the dough has doubled in size.

Step 2. Roll dough out with a rolling pin on a floured surface to a large rectangle about 50cm by 40cm.

Slice the butter and lay over half the dough and fold the dough over to cover the butter completely, press the edges together.

Roll dough out to about 40cm by 30cm, imagine the dough to be divided into three and fold each side into the middle.

Place on a floured tray and cover and leave to rest for 20 minutes

Step 3. Roll dough out to about 40cm by 30 cm, imagine the dough to be divided into three and fold each side into the middle.

Place on a floured tray and cover and leave to rest for 20 minutes

Step 4. Roll dough out to about 40cm by 30 cm, imagine the dough to be divided into three and fold each side into the middle.

Place on a floured tray and cover and leave to rest for 20 minutes or overnight.

Step 5. Early in the morning you want to bake your croissants.
Now we are ready to roll and shape the dough.

Roll the dough to a 20cm by 50cm rectangle and cut into 12 long triangles with the bases all equal sizes. Cut each base with a 3 cm slit in the middle of the base and roll up tightly from the split end and turn the edges in to make the croissants trademark crescent shape. Leave to rise in a warm place until doubled in size and bake in a hot 200°C oven for around 20 minutes until golden brown and cooked.

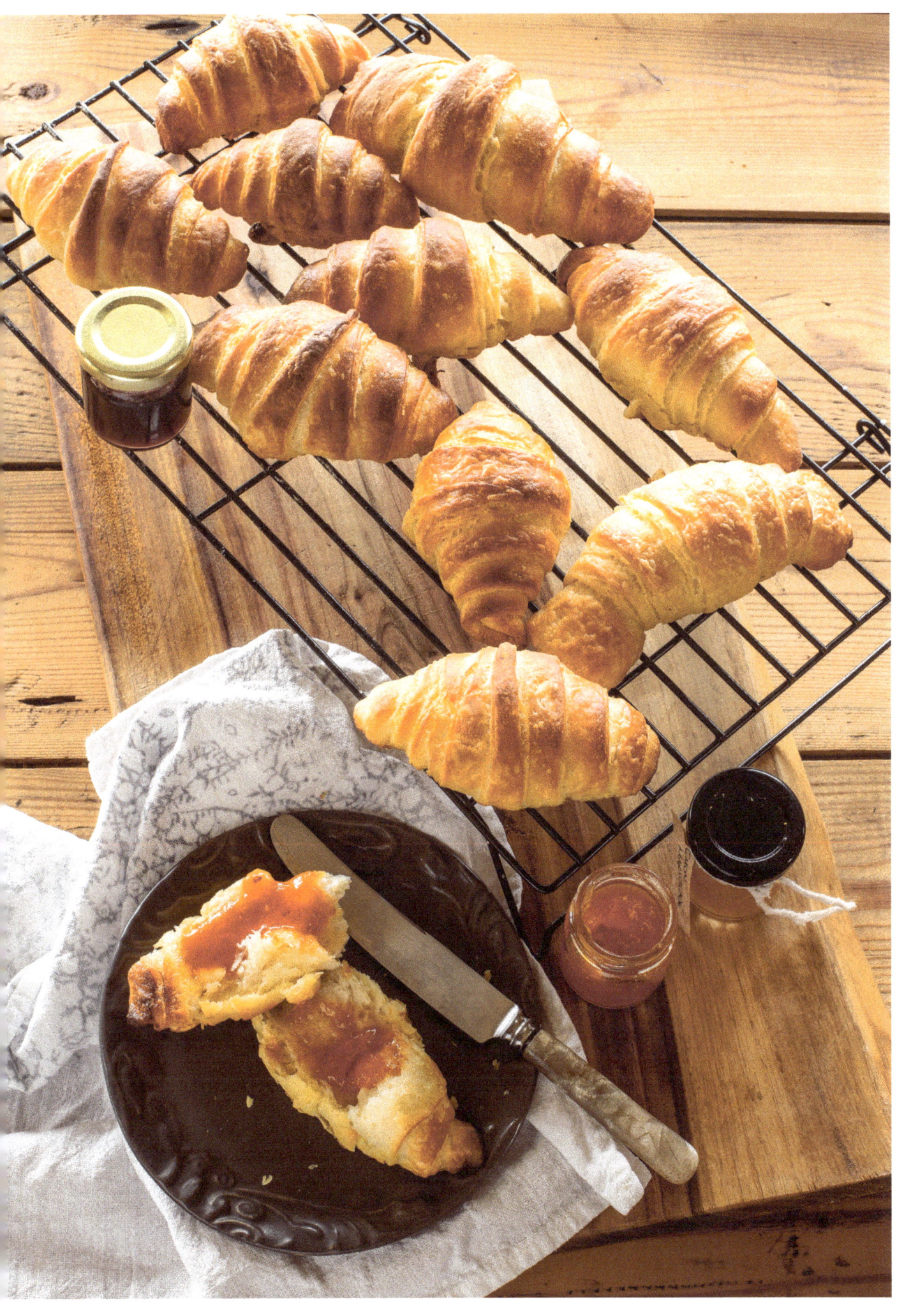

Blue Warhou Tartare

SERVES 4

Snotty trevally is another name for this fish, one of Tasmania's favourite fish. It is best consumed as close to catching as possible. When eaten raw or slightly cooked by this marinade, the fish is delicious. With a bit of prep, this dish is a super easy impressive dinner party entrée. Pick a big robust Tasmanian olive oil such as Freshfield Grove's Picual for this dish to match the big flavours from the vinegar and pickles.

400 grams blue warhou skinless, boneless fillets

2 tablespoons capers

2 large gherkins

1 tablespoon dill

pinch sea salt

50ml red wine vinegar

50ml lemon juice

50ml robust extra virgin olive oil

Slice and dice the fish into a 5mm dice. Dice the gherkins and cut the capers if large into a 2mm dice. Pick the dill into small pieces.

Mix the fish, dill, capers, juice from the lemon, gherkin and vinegar in a bowl and arrange on 4 plates. Finish with a drizzle of the olive oil.

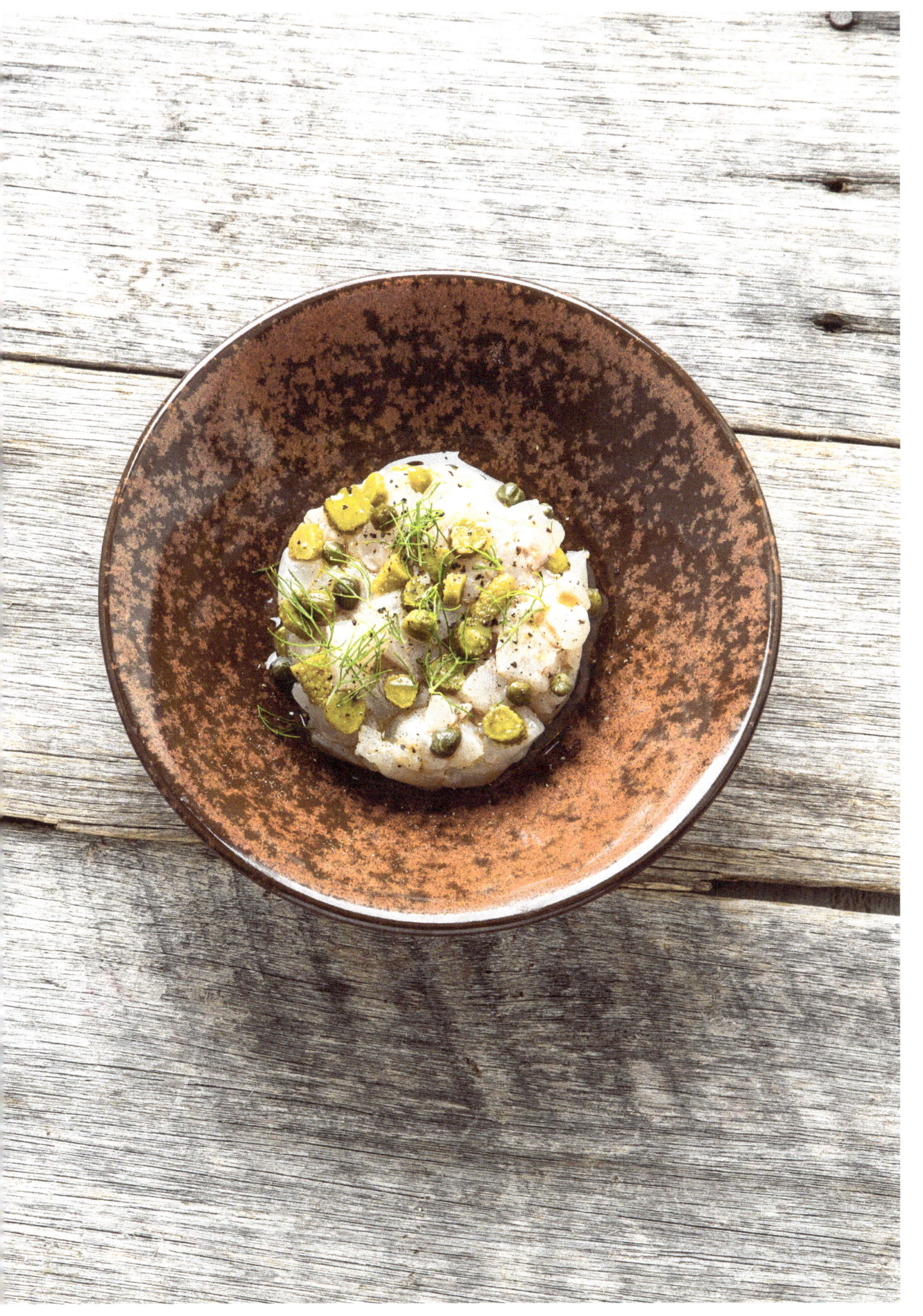

Baked Quince and Blue Cheese with Vino Cotto

SERVES 4

This recipe is always an absolute hit in my workshops and Indulgence weekends. Its a beautiful recipe created when I had a truckload of quinces from my trees. After I had made plenty of quince paste, quince jelly, created a savoury barbeque sauce, bottled heaps and cooked every sweet dessert with quinces imaginable, I needed a savoury idea for my menus. Use a creamy rich blue cheese such as the King Island Roaring Forties blue. Bake the quinces when fresh and then during winter use bottled and preserved quinces with a shorter baking time. Add some smoked quail, venison or crusty sourdough to turn this decadent entrée into a fancy lunch or dinner, or on the side of a grilled pork chop or beef steak to jazz up a weeknight meal.

extra virgin olive oil

2 large quinces

200 grams Roaring Forties blue

100ml vino cotto

Heat the oven to 180°C.

Cut the quinces into 8 pieces and remove the pips and hard area around the pips. Place the pieces skin side down in a baking dish and drizzle with the olive oil, bake in the oven for about 30 minutes or until the quinces are soft.

When using the preserved quinces simply place in the oven for a few minutes, long enough for them to heat through. Spread the cheese on top and place the tray back in the oven for 10 minutes.

Drizzle with vino cotto and serve.

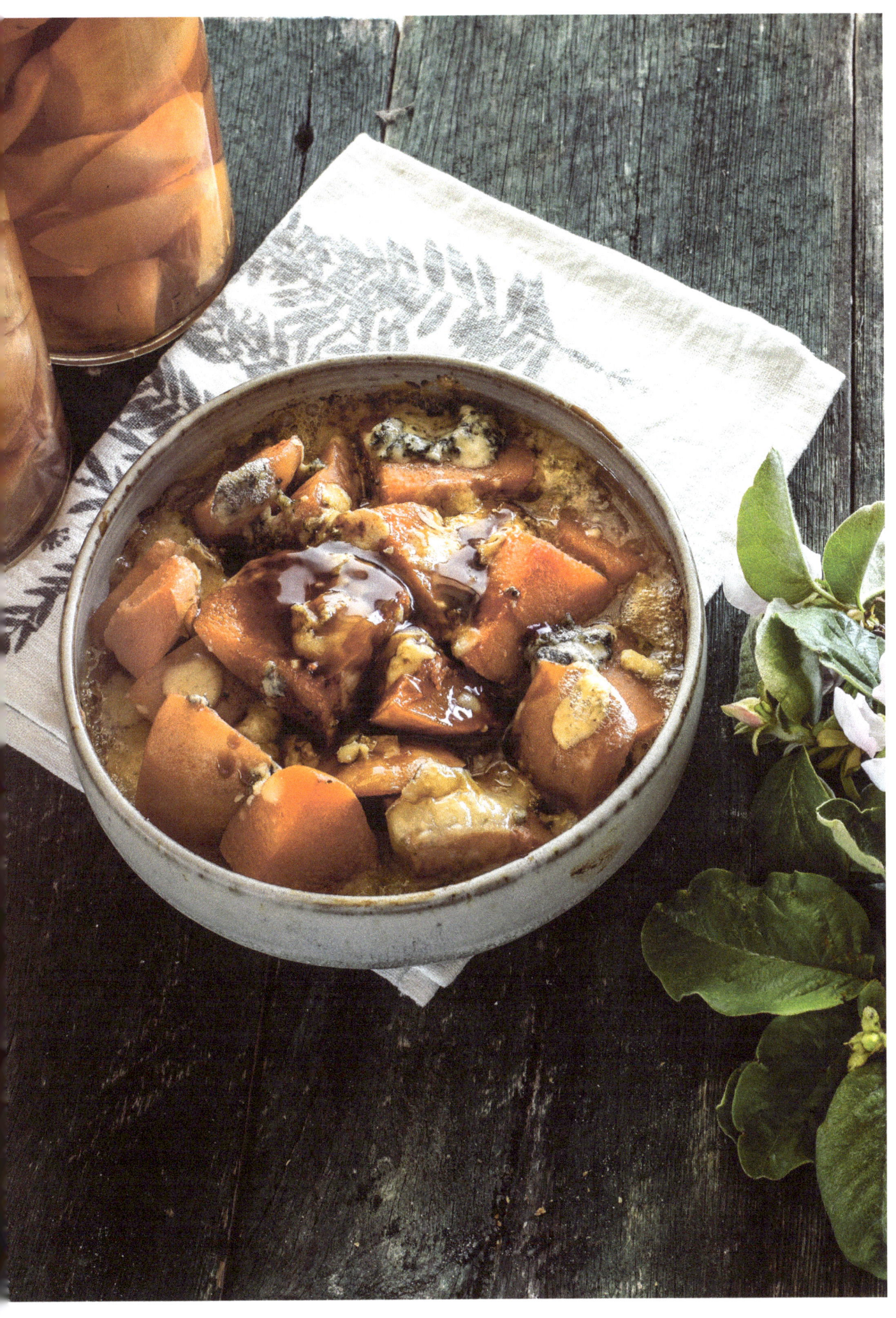

Cabbage Rolls

MAKES 8-12 LARGE ROLLS

Don't be shy to use some of the outer leaves for these rolls. I normally discard anything that's a bit tough and rough. But if you pinch a bit of the outer leaf and if it tastes OK and not bitter or tough, then it is perfectly fine to use. For the filling preferably use handfuls of fresh aromatic herbs such as oregano, sage, thyme, rosemary, parsley and basil that you have in your garden, but a simple Italian mix of oregano and basil will suffice if using dried herbs from the pantry.

1 large cabbage

300 grams Summerlea farm beef mince

2 onions

1 leek

4 cloves garlic

2 medium zucchini

2 large carrots

4 tablespoons herbs, dry parsley, basil and oregano will do

100 grams long grain rice

FOR THE SAUCE

800 grams tomato chopped or puréed. A tin will do

2 large onions

6 cloves garlic

50ml robust extra virgin olive oil

300ml stock (chicken, beef or veg)

2 tablespoons basil

2 tablespoons oregano

salt

pepper

Heat the oven to 180°C.

To prepare the cabbage leaves bring a large pot of water to the boil. Carefully peel the leaves of the cabbage off and cut out the hard centre stalk of each leaf. Blanch the leaves in the boiling water for about 30 seconds or until soft. Drain and cool, lay out on the bench.

To prepare the filling, in a large bowl mix the mince, finely diced onion, finely diced leek, crushed garlic, grated zucchini, carrot and chopped herbs. Add the rice that has been washed a few times by putting it in a sieve and running under water.

To make the sauce, in a large heavy based pan sauté the finely diced onions and crushed garlic until soft in the olive oil. Add the tomato, chicken stock, basil and oregano and season well with salt and pepper. Cook for around 20 minutes until cooked and flavoursome.

Add the mince mixture to the cabbage leaves, in the middle of each leaf, so it's evenly distributed. Roll up each cabbage roll with the fold underneath. Lay the cabbage rolls in a baking dish and cover with the tomato sauce.

Bake the cabbage rolls for around 40 minutes in a 180°C oven until the mince is cooked through and the rice is cooked is almost cooked.

Leave to rest covered to continue cooking for at least 20 minutes and serve crumbled with feta. They are also a delicious cold lunch.

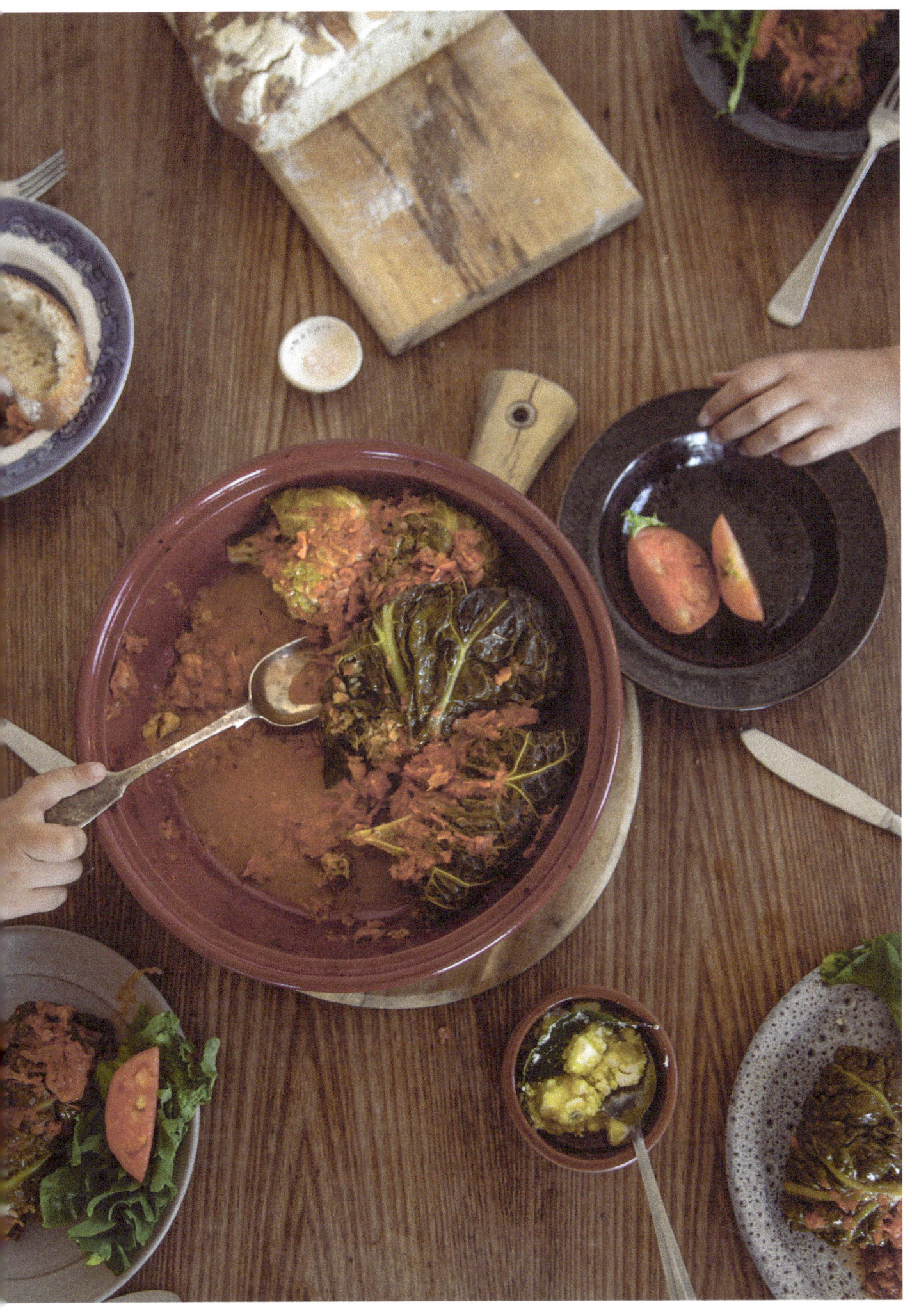

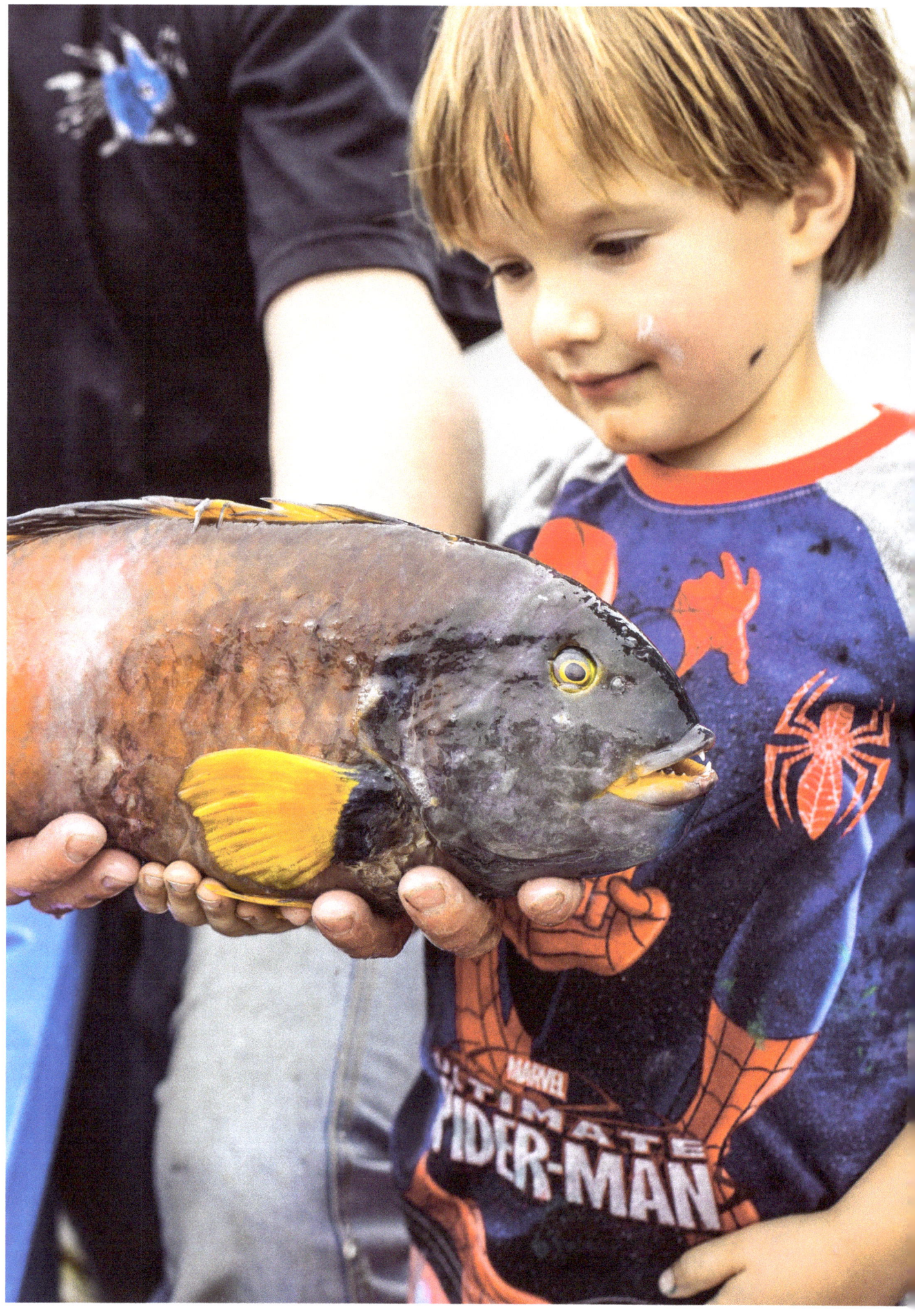

"My children are fascinated by where thier food comes from. They have learnt to respect food, and appreciate who has grown or farmed it. I'm hoping as adults this will help them make good choices."

Beetroot Wellington

SERVES 12

Find the recipe to make your own puff pastry on my website, www.eloiseemmett.com

Otherwise a store bought pastry is a quicker option to this stunning special occasion meat free meal.

8 medium beetroots

5 sheets puff pastry

100 grams marinated feta

1 brown onion

4 cloves garlic

2 cups spinach

2 kohlrabi (or use cabbage)

2 bunches of herbs that go well with veggies a mix of rosemary, thyme, basil, parsley, tarragon, oregano and chervil.

salt

pepper

extra virgin olive oil

egg for egg wash (a leftover egg white or yolk you've frozen will do)

Heat the oven to 180°C.

Place the washed beetroot in a baking tray and roll in the olive oil and bake for 30 minutes or until soft to poke with a skewer. Cool and peel the beetroot.

Meanwhile peel and crush garlic and slice the onion, finely dice kohlrabi if using and slice spinach and pick and roughly chop herbs. In a large heavy based pan sauté onion, garlic and kohlrabi in olive oil. Mix through, spinach and herbs so they wilt slightly and cool.

Lay four sheets of pastry out to make a large square, by overlapping the sheets by 1cm, stick the sheets together with the egg wash and press together.

Lay the cooled onion mix in the centre of the large square of pastry in a strip as wide as your beetroot, this is making a base to lay your beetroot on, leaving the ends free of mix. Lay the beetroots down the middle and then add the marinated feta.

Fold the ends of the pastry in and roll to seal, trying to be aware of any thick clumps of pastry that will not cook through, so the pastry is even all over. Keep the top the lightest place in pastry, as we have reserved the last sheet to create a lattice on top.

With the last sheet of pastry, create a lattice pattern on top for a unique finish. View my website for details.

Bake in an oven for 40 minutes or until golden brown all over and cooked through.

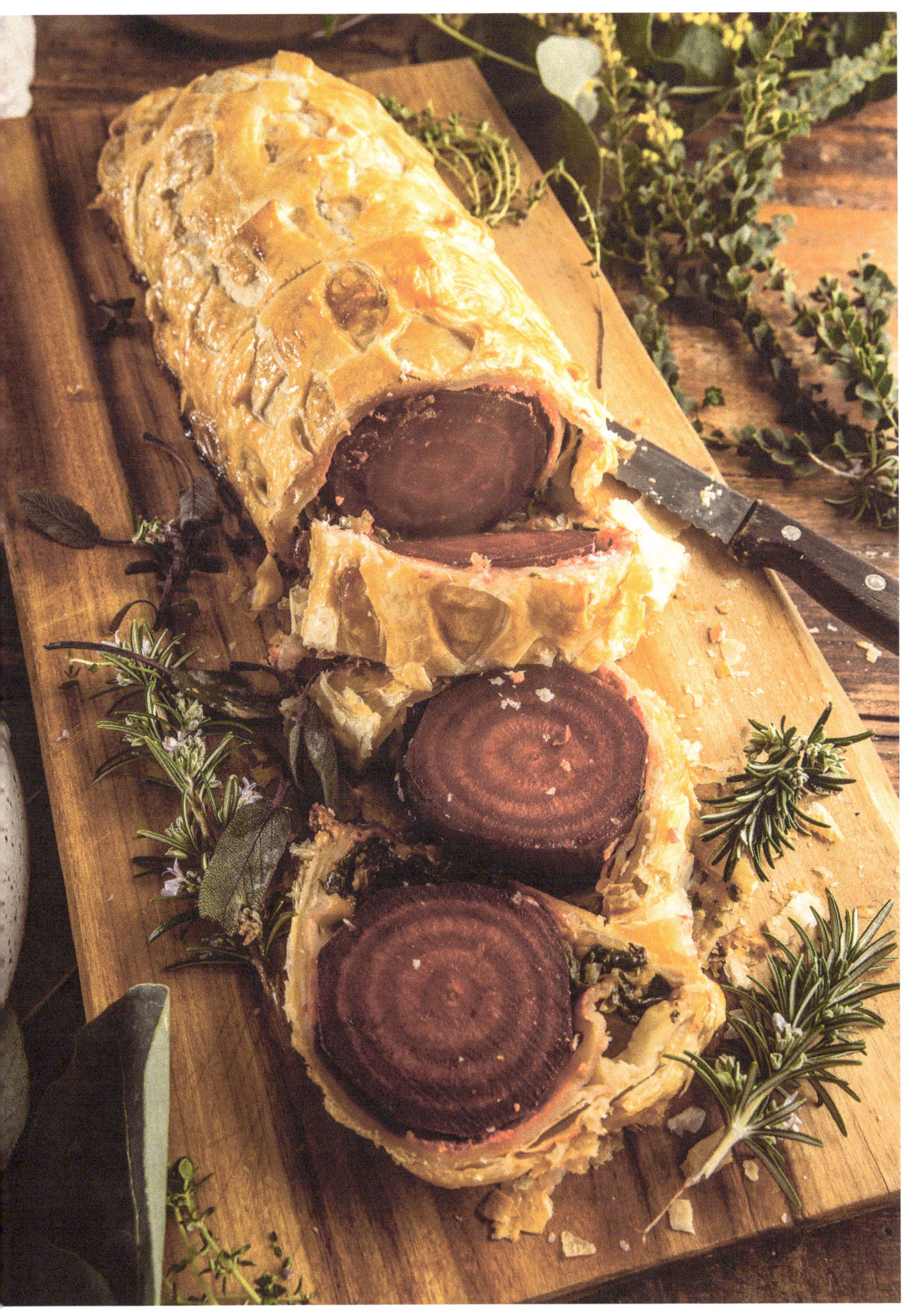

Lenah Game Meats Wallaby Fillet with Goats Cheese and Cherry Chutney

SERVES 4

Wallaby is an excellent source of protein and is also low in fat. I make this chutney in bulk with cherry seconds from the Port Arthur Cherry Farm and I serve it with wallaby, quail and venison though out the year. This recipe is enough for a small jar to store in the fridge for 2 or 3 meals. The wallaby can be simply tossed on the barbeque and is best served cooked medium rare and rested after cooking. The low fat content of the meat will make it tough if cooked for too long.

4 Lenah Game Meats Wallaby fillets approximately 120 grams each

800 grams pumpkin

extra virgin olive oil

100 grams goats cheese

100 grams spinach leaves

CHERRY CHUTNEY

1 tablespoon extra virgin olive oil

200 grams cherries

1 small red onion

2 tablespoons vinegar

2 tablespoons brown sugar

Heat the oven to 180°C.

To make the chutney, peel and finely dice the onion and sauté in a pot with the extra virgin olive oil until soft. Add the halved and pitted cherries and vinegar and simmer until cooked and the sugar until the chutney has reduced and thickened.

Peel and chop the pumpkin into chunky 2cm pieces and place them in a baking dish with a drizzle of extra virgin olive oil, bake for about 30 minutes until cooked just before serving. While the pumpkin is still hot, toss through the picked and washed spinach leaves and goats cheese.

Leave the wallaby out of the fridge for an hour before cooking. To cook the wallaby brush with extra virgin olive oil and grill on a medium high heat on the barbeque or the frying pan on the stove. Depending on the size of the fillets but for an average fillet it will take around 8 minutes turning a few times. Wrap in foil to rest for 10 minutes before slicing and serving with the salad and chutney.

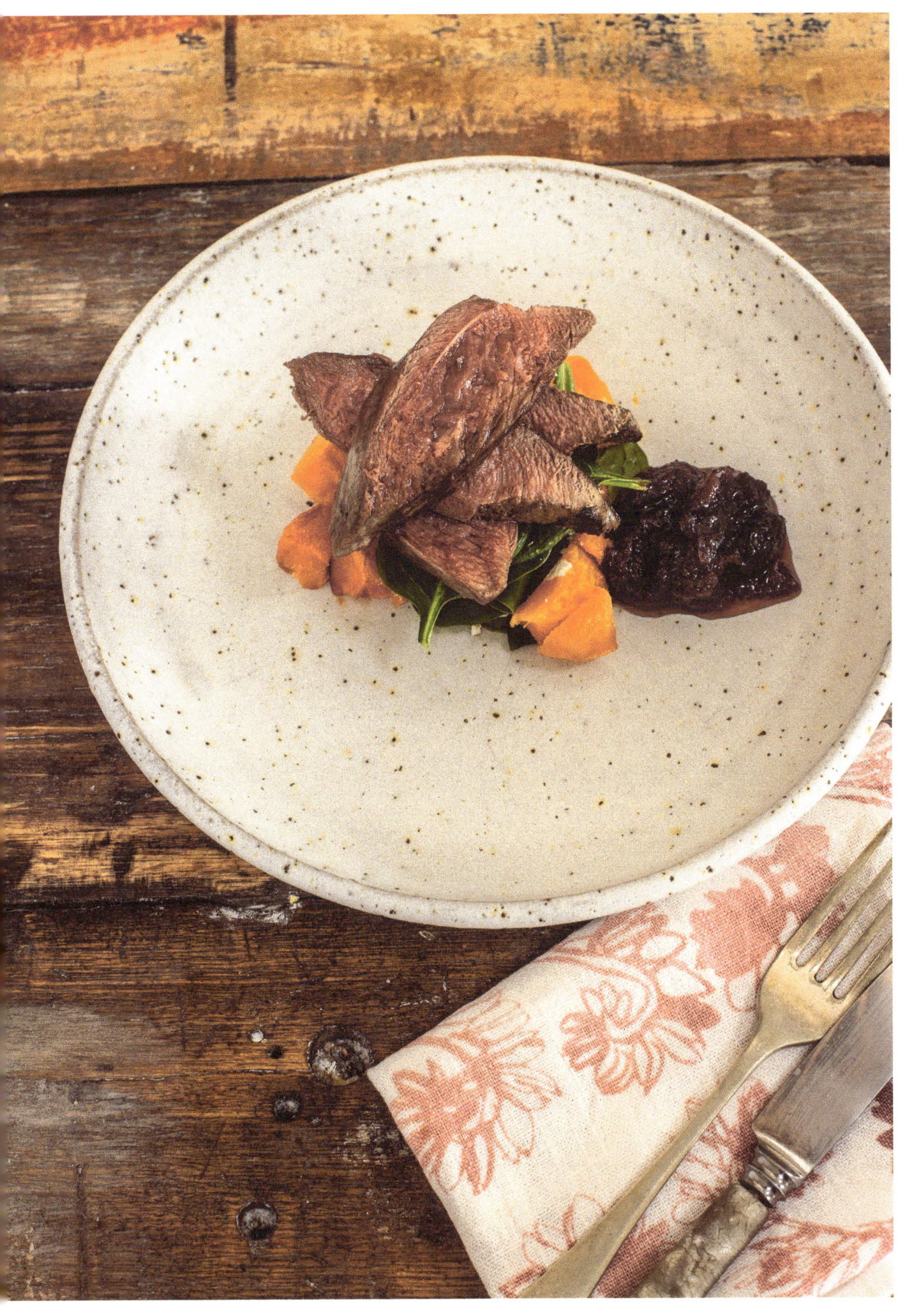

Hot and Sour Wakame and Cameron of Tasmania Oysters Broth

SERVES 4

Oysters are little balls of nutrition. As lovely as it is to quaff a dozen with some champagne, you only need to consume three for all the amazing nutritional benefits. If you have a stash of good quality stocks in the freezer, this is a simple and delicious quick meal! Alternatively you can purchase a pre-made stock such as Mures fish stock.

1 dozen Cameron of Tasmania pacific oysters

1 litre fish stock

100 grams wakame dried or fresh

bunch of bok choy

½ long red chilli

1 tablespoon sesame oil

2 tablespoons ponzu

2 spring onions

1 teaspoon ginger

juice of one lemon

juice of one lime

200 grams udon noodles

Finely slice the ginger, chilli and spring onions into thin strips. Heat a large heavy based pan to a medium high heat and fry the shallots and ginger add the stock and bring to the boil.

Wash and cut the wakame and bok choy into bite size chunks and add to the pot, add the ponzu and juices and season with salt and pepper add the noodles and serve.

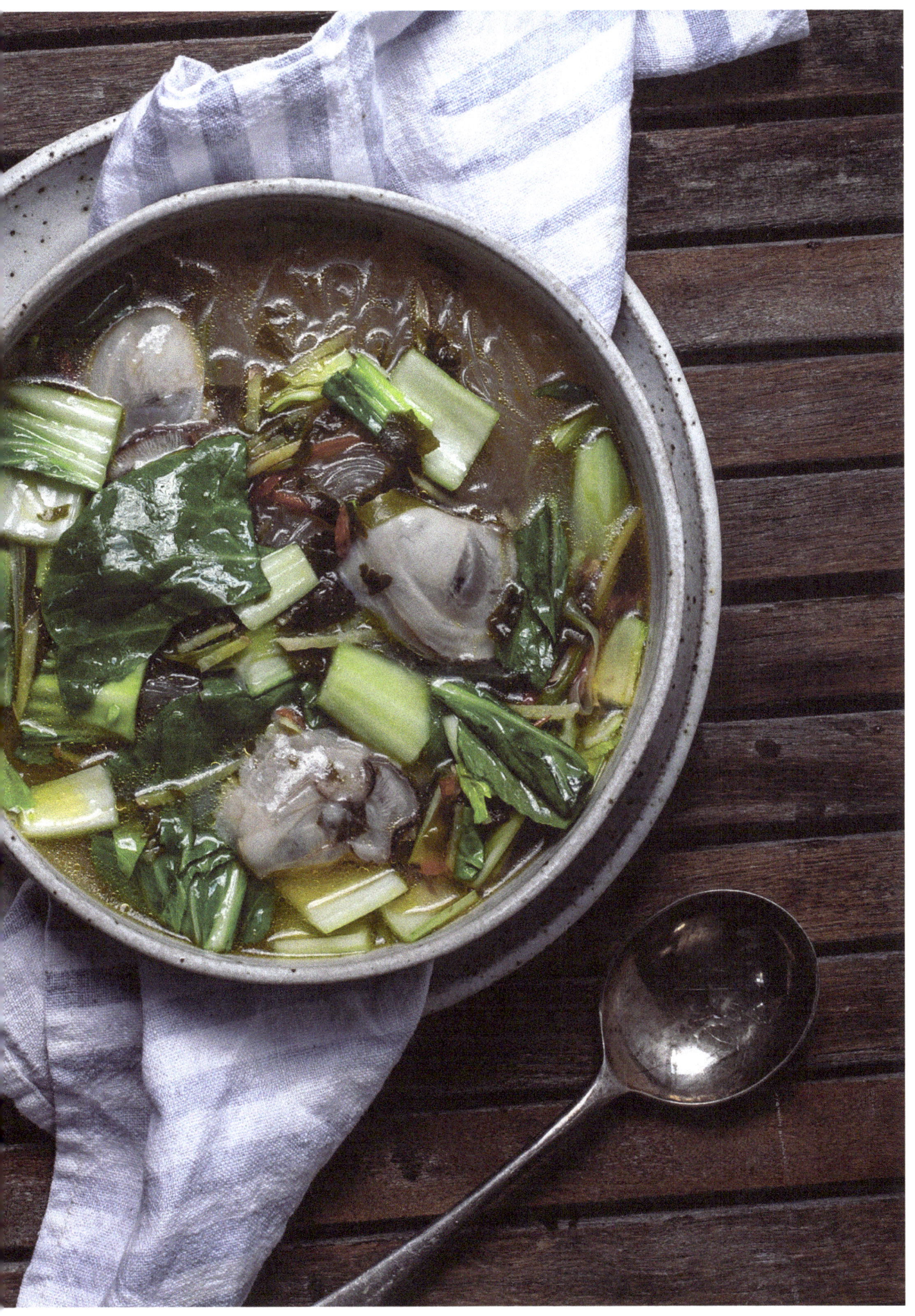

Blue Cheese Arancini

SERVES 6-8 FOR ENTREE

RISOTTO RICE

1 onion

3 cloves garlic

1 tablespoon extra virgin olive oil

150 grams arborio rice

100ml white wine

200ml chicken stock

40 grams parmesan

100 grams blue cheese

200 grams flour

1 egg

200ml milk

100 grams breadcrumbs

robust extra virgin olive oil for deep frying

AIOLI

egg

1 clove garlic

1 tablespoon white vinegar

extra virgin olive oil

salt

pepper

To make the risotto rice, finely dice the onion and crush the garlic and fry them in a heavy based pan with the extra virgin olive oil. Add the rice and sauté for a minute or two and then the stock and wine, simmer while stirring until the rice is just cooked through, this will take around 15 minutes. Lay out in a thin layer on a tray to cool in the refrigerator.

When the rice is cool transfer to a bowl, add the cheese and mix well. Shape and press into firm balls around the size of a twenty-cent piece in diameter. Put the balls on a tray and put back in the fridge to stay cold.

Make an egg wash by cracking the egg and mixing with the milk. Put the flour in a separate bowl and the bread crumbs in a third bowl. Then dip each ball into the flour, then the egg and then the breadcrumb, shaking excess flour, egg wash, or crumbs off as you go.

To deep fry, fill a deep heavy based pan with extra virgin olive oil to about 3cm deep. Heat to 170°C and fry the balls rolling them to make sure they are evenly cooked and brown all over.

Extra virgin olive oil can handle 6 hours of cooking before it starts to lose its nutritional value so don't chuck it out when you are finished cooking. Drain any remaining oil and store in the fridge (as its now contaminated and could go off easier, use it to cook your barbeque, eggs, fish and more in the next few days). The fresh herb flavours will dull in the first cooking but it remains clean in cooking without that foul rancid deep fryer smell and taste we are all accustomed too.

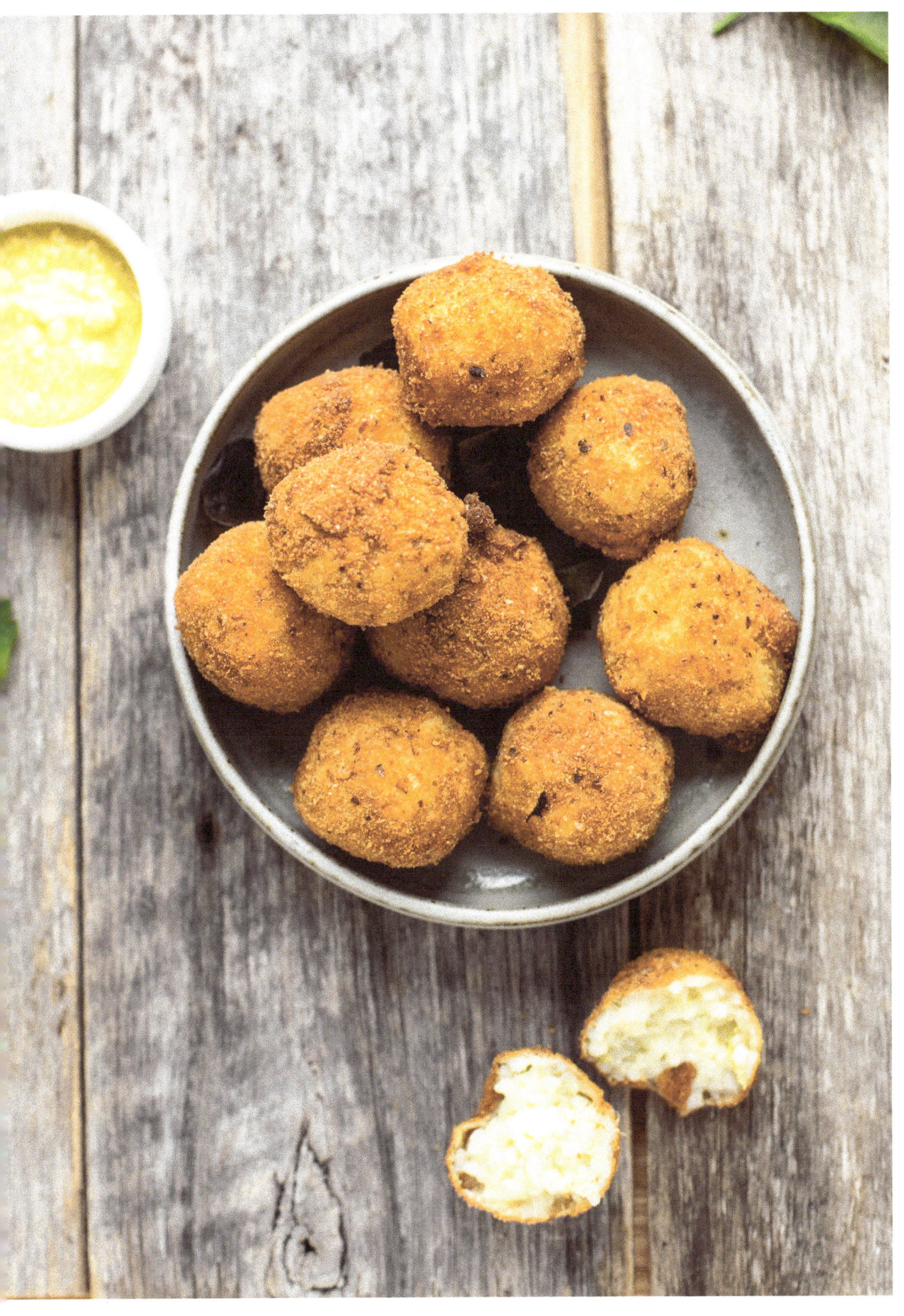

Quail Roasted with Bacon and Tarragon with Garlic Roast Pink Eyes and Green Beans

SERVES 4

I think we all love a fancy delicious one pan dinner party meal for ease of serving when we have guests. This quail dish also works well in a camp oven if you desire something a bit posh while camping.

4 partially boned quail

4 rashers bacon

1 tablespoon extra virgin olive oil

6 cloves garlic

1 red onion

8 small pinkeye potatoes

4 long sprigs tarragon

2 teaspoons butter

salt and pepper

400 grams green beans

Heat the oven to 180°C.

To prepare the quail rub both sides with butter, and season with a sprinkle of salt and pepper, wrap the quail up in bacon with the tarragon between the skin of the quail and the bacon.

Peel the garlic, leave the cloves whole, peel and cut the onion into large wedges, and place these on the base of a heavy base baking tray with the extra virgin olive oil. Scrub the pinkeye potatoes and add them to the pan. Trim both ends of the green beans.

Bake for about 35 minutes. Throw the green beans in the tray with a good splash of extra virgin olive oil after about 30 minutes, for the last 5 minutes to cook them.

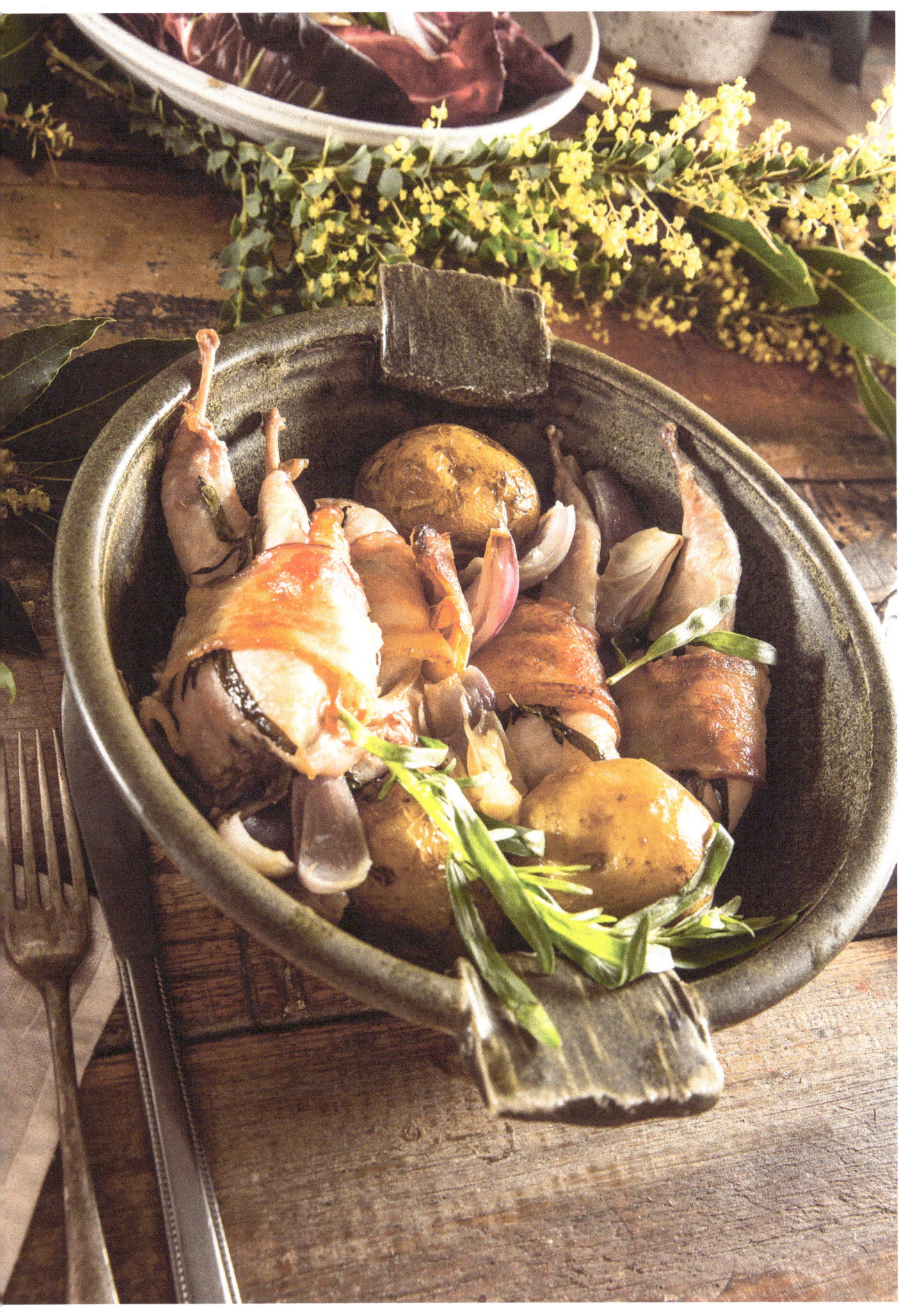

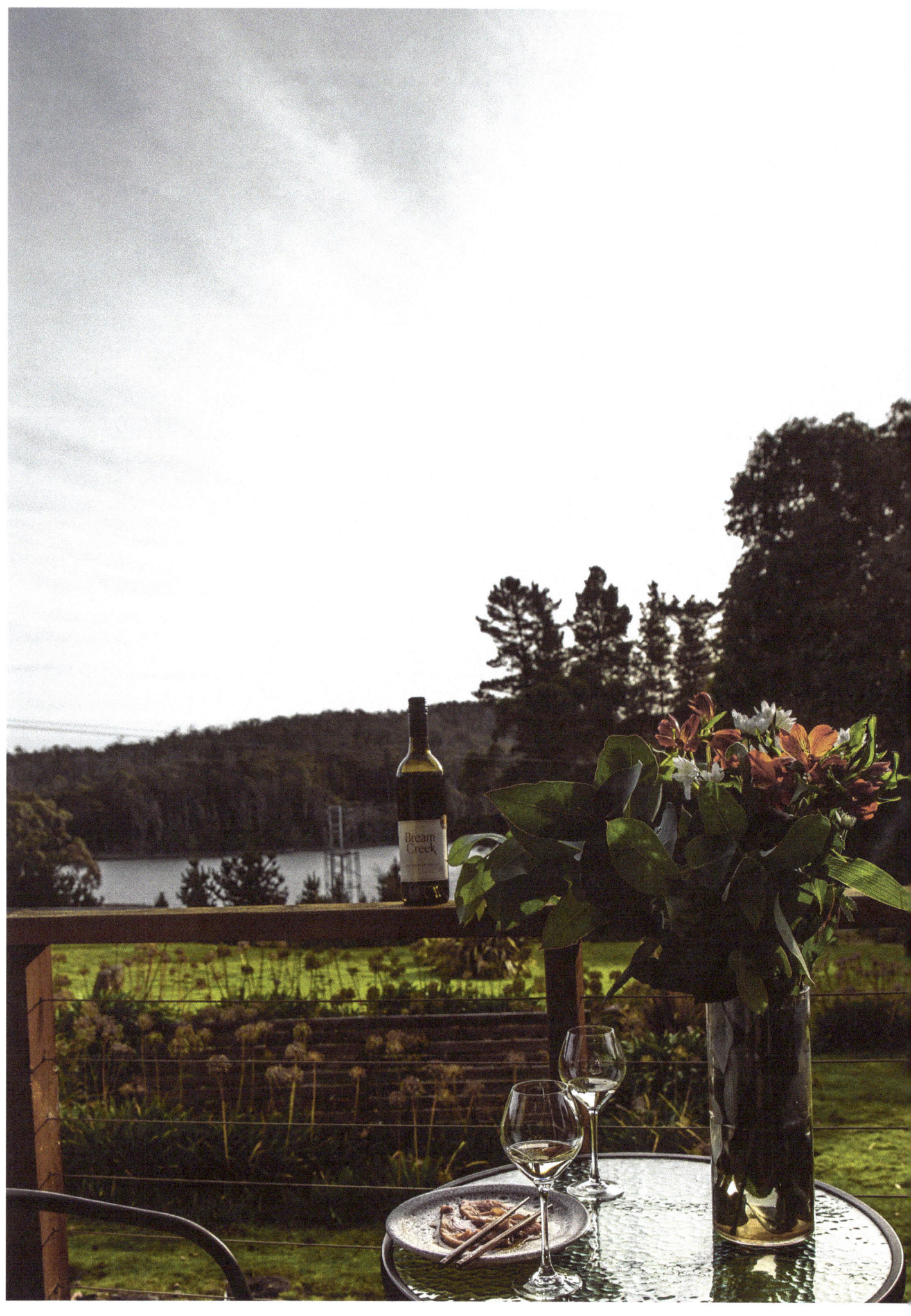

"I am aware about my mindset around cooking – Instead of thinking that cooking is a chore, I instead feel blessed to be able to feed my family well."

Quince, Lavender and Freshfield Grove Extra Virgin Olive Oil Cake

SERVES 12

Recipe by Fiona Makowski

If you haven't baked a cake with extra virgin olive oil then you really must! Delicious. This versatile recipe can be used with or without lavender and any fruit you like, if using fresh quince then they would need to be stewed until pink and cooked and cooled before assembling in the cake batter. This is a fancy cake for morning tea at Little Norfolk Bay workshops, but also my boy Oscar's favourite lunchbox treat.

80ml Freshfield Grove extra virgin olive oil

1 teaspoon culinary lavender

80 grams sugar

½ teaspoon vanilla

2 eggs

1 teaspoon lemon zest

50ml milk

160 grams self-raising flour

pinch salt

3 bottled quinces

Heat the oven to 180°C.

Line a 20cm spring form tin, or your favourite serving flan dish with baking paper or oil and flour.

In your mixer, blender or a bowl beat the olive oil, lavender and sugar well until creamy. Beat in the eggs, vanilla, lemon zest and milk. Beat in self raising flour and salt and pour the batter into the prepared cake tin.

Drain and slice the quince and lay on top.

Bake in the 180°C oven for around 25 minutes until cooked through. Test to see if the cake is cooked by poking with a skewer and if it comes out clean (without any raw cake batter) it is ready.

Remove the cake from the tin if using the tin and serve cool, warm or cold.

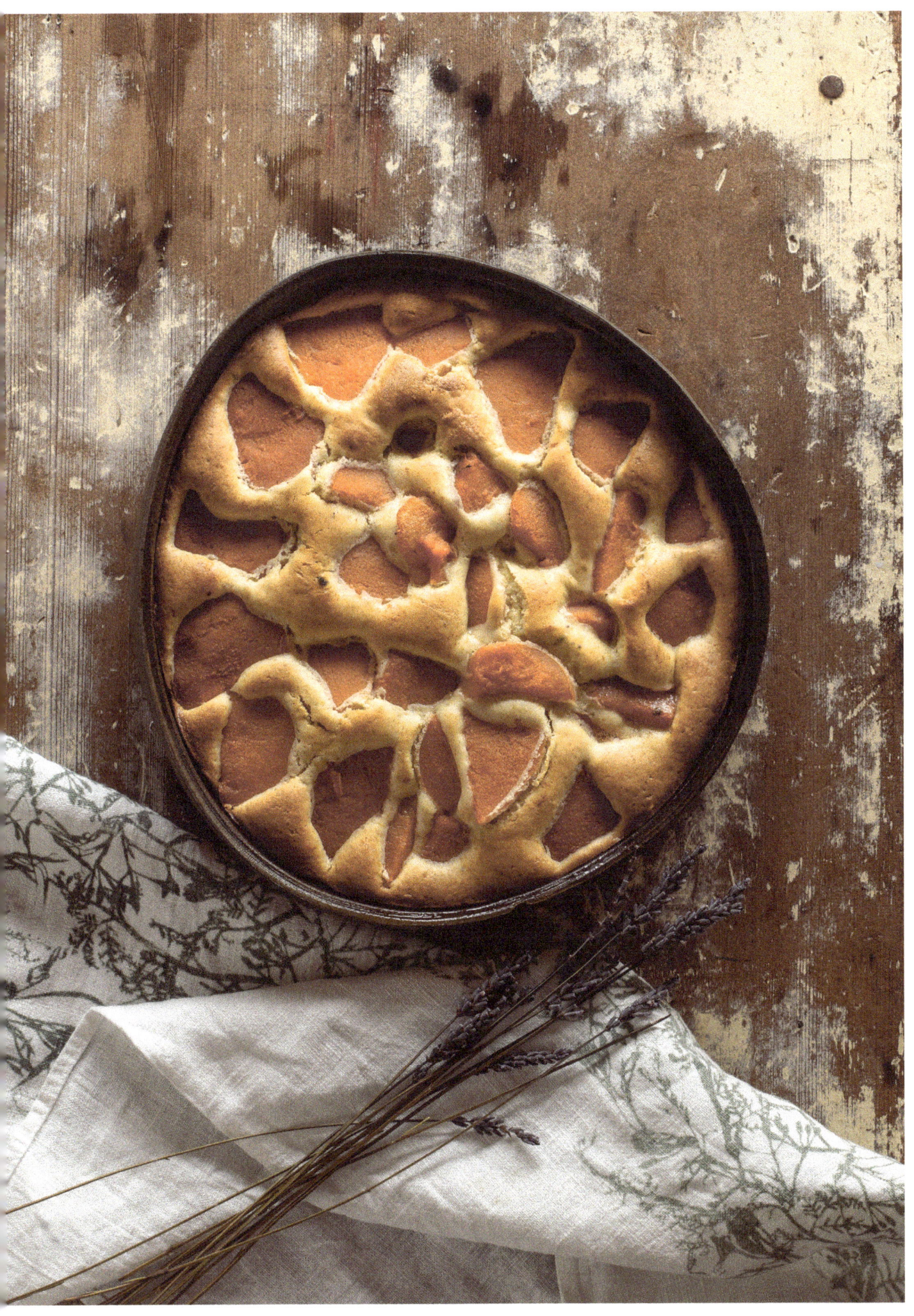

Hazelnut and Green Peppercorn Crusted Lamb with Lost Pipin Cider and Apple Risotto

SERVES 4

4 x 4 point lamb racks

CRUST

1 tablespoon green peppercorns

4 tablespoons hazelnuts

4 slices bread

2 cloves garlic

2 sprigs rosemary

2 tablespoons butter

RISOTTO

3 cloves garlic

1 onion

1 tablespoon olive oil

2 apples

200 grams arborio rice

200ml beef stock

375ml Lost Pipin cider

80 grams parmesan cheese

100ml cream

2 handfuls spinach

sea salt

pepper

SAUCE

375ml beef stock

375ml Lost Pipin cider

Heat the oven to 180°C.

To prepare the lamb trim visible fat and sinew. In a food processor blitz the bread into crumbs and place in a bowl. Blitz the nuts, garlic, rosemary and butter to create a smooth paste. Mix the paste through the crumbs well and divide into four and press firmly onto each rack.

Lay baking paper on a baking tray and lay the racks crust side down and bake in the oven for around 20 minutes (depending on size and fat content) to achieve a medium doneness. Wrap in kitchen foil and rest for at least 10 minutes.

To make the risotto, crush the garlic and finely dice the onion and sauté them in a heavy based pan with the oil until translucent. Add the rice and continue sautéing for one minute and then add the finely chopped apple, stock and the cider. Once it has come back to the boil, reduce the heat to a gentle simmer and continue to stir regularly until the rice is cooked through. Add the cream, cheese and spinach until heated and cooked and season with salt and pepper and serve.

To make the sauce reduce the stock and cider in a heavy based pan by simmering gently until the sauce is around a third of the original volume. Season with sea salt and pepper.

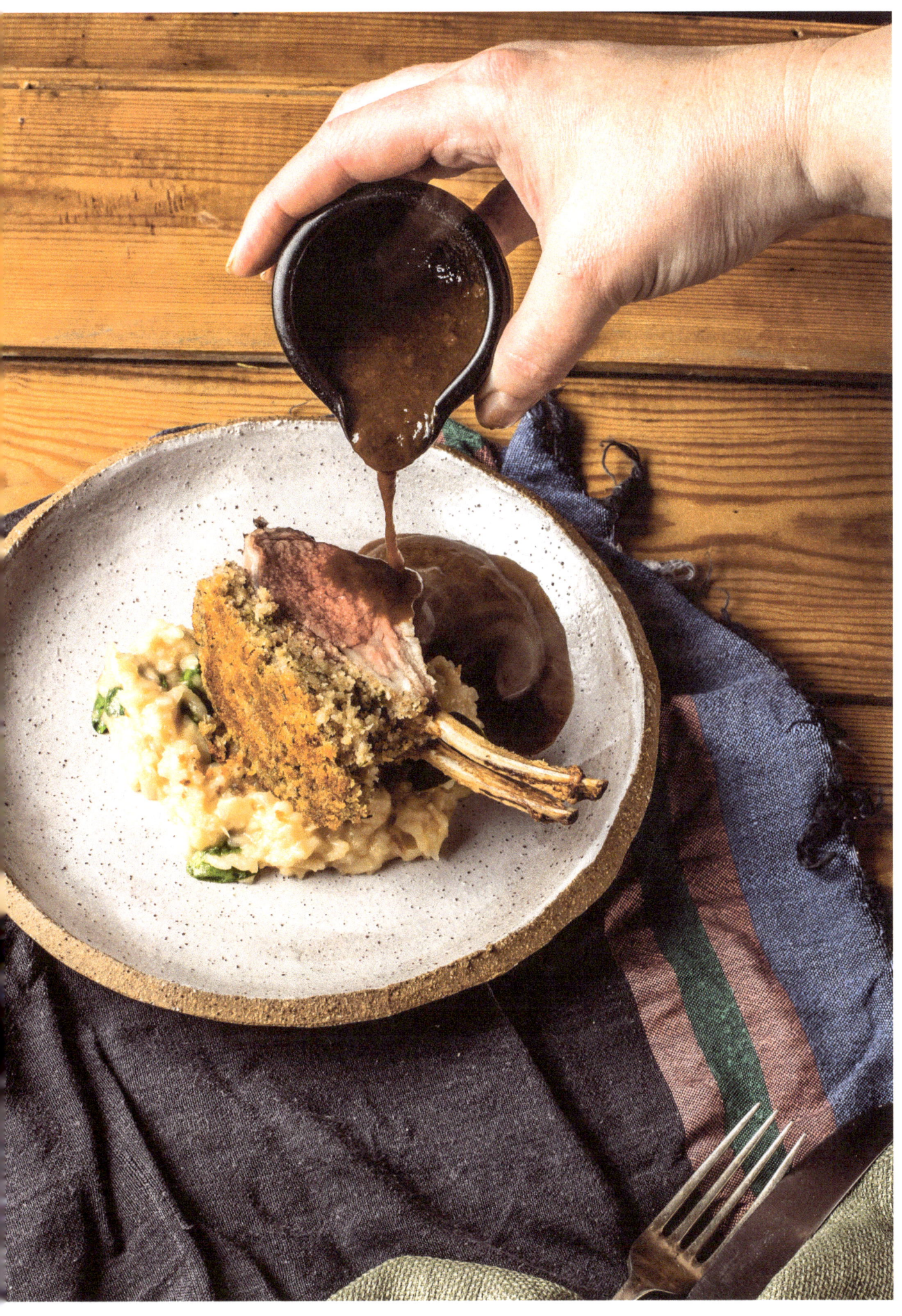

FREYCINET MARINE FARM

Chorizo, Chilli, Freycinet Marine Farm Mussels and Handmade Pasta

SERVES 4

If you've pre-made or are using store bought pasta then this dish is super easy and quick to whip up. I will always make my own pasta for a special dish like this, you cannot beat the taste of homemade pasta.

extra virgin olive oil

1 long red chilli

1 onion

4 cloves garlic

800 grams tomatoes

1 chorizo sausage

2 tablespoons basil

2 tablespoons oregano

sea salt

cracked black pepper

300 grams fresh pasta cut into fettuccine (see page 96 for recipe)

1 kilo live mussels

100ml white wine

The sauce can be prepared earlier, even a day or two before to let the flavours infuse. Finely dice the garlic, onion and chilli and sauté in the olive oil in a heavy based pan. Add the chorizo sausage that has been peeled and diced into a 3mm dice. Add the finely chopped or crushed tomato and herbs, season with salt and pepper and simmer for 25 minutes.

Bring a large pot of water to the boil - the pasta will only take a few minutes to cook so be ready to place the pasta it in the pot when the mussels are nearly cooked. As soon as you start to cook your mussels put the pasta in to cook and drain, ready to toss through the sauce.

To cook the mussels, heat a large pan until hot, throw in the mussels and the wine for a minute and then the sauce stirring well The mussels will only take a few minutes to cook - they are pretty much cooked when they have opened. Taking care not to overcook the mussels - when most of the mussels have opened toss through the pasta and serve immediately. If you have a stubborn mussel that didn't open simply prize it open with a knife.

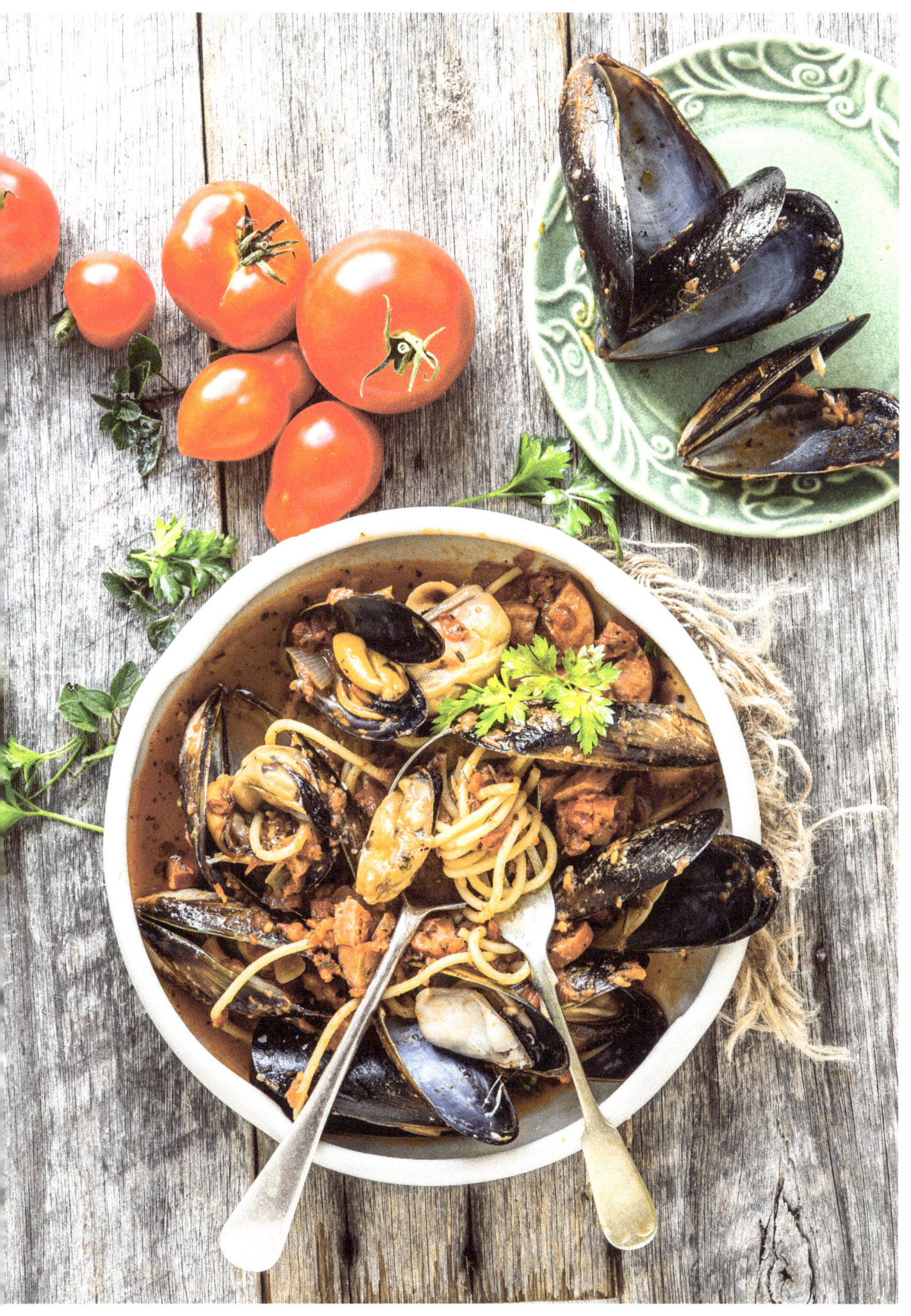

Spiced Cauliflower and Labneh

SERVES 4

Labneh is a great introduction to the process of cheese making that anyone can simply do at home. It is a delicious refrigerator staple used to heighten the flavours of simple food. Although it is best to roast and grind your spices when you are going to need them, making a few tablespoons extra and freezing them makes for a very easy tasty meal, on any veggie.

500ml natural yogurt

1 teaspoon salt

robust extra virgin olive oil such as Freshfield Grove Picul

1 teaspoon turmeric

1 teaspoon coriander

1 teaspoon cumin

1 teaspoon garam masala

½ teaspoon pepper

½ teaspoon cayenne

1 teaspoon fennel

1 teaspoon sea salt

1 teaspoon pepper

1 cup flour

1 egg

TO SERVE

rocket or greens

To make the labneh, mix the natural yogurt and salt together and sit in a cheesecloth over a bowl in the fridge or sink for a few hours to strain. Keep the liquid (refrigerate or freeze if you need) to put in your next loaf of bread so it is not wasted. Once quite firm transfer to a container and refrigerate.

Place your spices into a pan and gently roast over a low heat until they are fragrant. When cool, finely grind and store any leftovers in a tightly sealed container in the freezer.

Slice the cauliflower into 7mm steaks. Mix 3 teaspoons spice mix with 3 tablespoons flour. Crack and whisk egg. Dip each piece of cauliflower into the egg then the spiced flour.

Heat the oil in a heavy based pan over a low to medium heat and fry each piece until golden brown and cooked through.

Serve the labneh, cauliflower and rocket with a good splash of the extra virgin olive oil and sea salt.

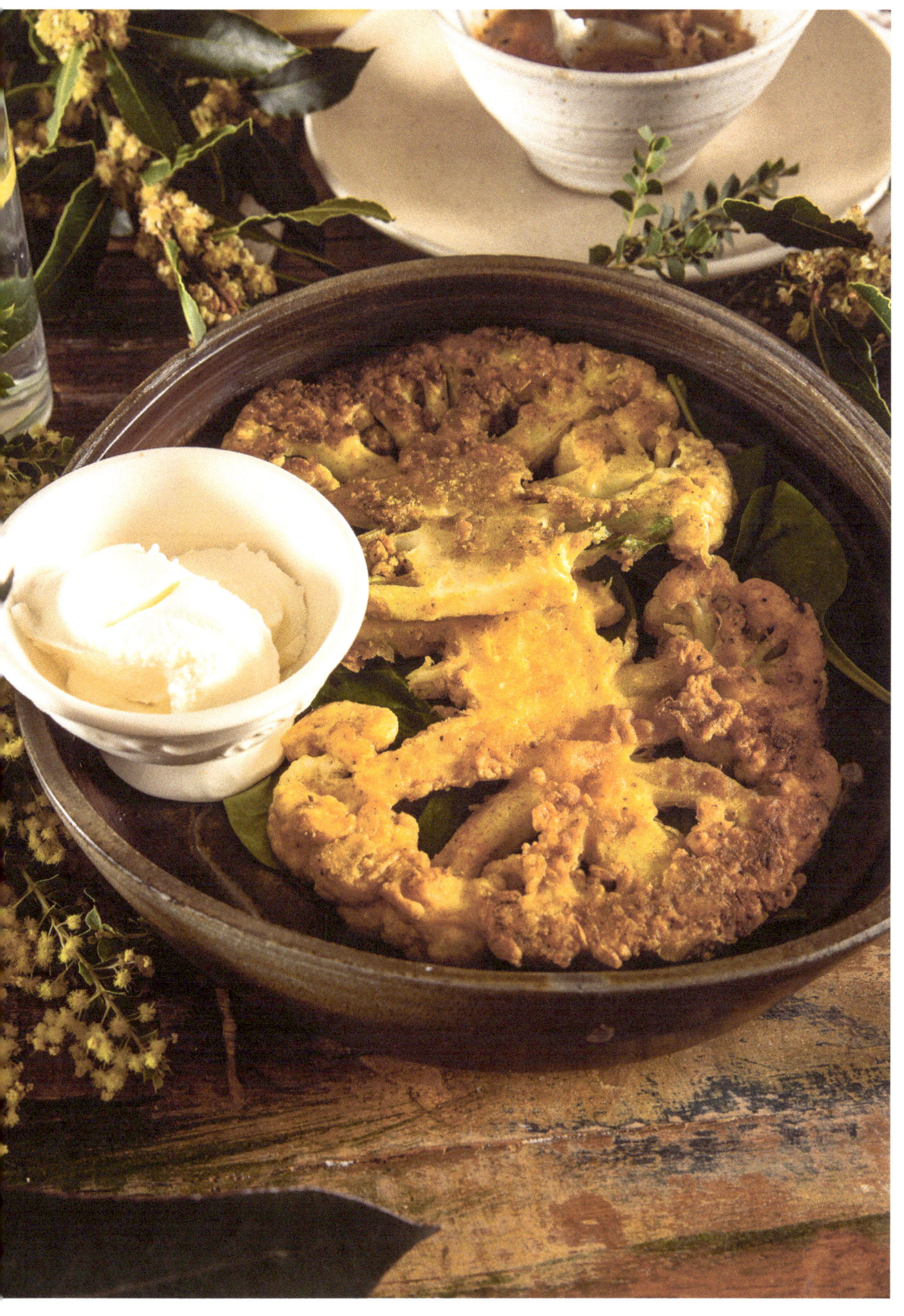

Sautéed Lentil Stuffed Tomato

SERVES 6

When tomatoes are in season they really need to be the hero of the dish. Oddly, coriander is a nice herb to suit this sautéed lentil stuffing, however a nice handful of and fresh herbs from your garden, freezer or pantry such as parsley, thyme, sage, rosemary, chives, will do. Many variations and combinations of this dish have appeared on my menus over the years, and still do. This exact version was complimented as the best vegetarian dish a vegetarian had ever eaten back in my days cooking as a chef de partie on Bedarra Island. If blue cheese is not your thing then a strong cheddar or parmesan also works well in the sauce.

STUFFED TOMATOES

6 ripe tomatoes (pretty much any variety will do)

100 grams lentils (soaked and cooked or from the tin)

1 medium onion

2 cloves garlic

salt and pepper

1 tablespoon butter

handful aromatic herbs

robust extra virgin olive oil

POLENTA

100 grams polenta

1 onion

1 clove garlic

1 tablespoon butter

100 grams mushrooms

500mls milk

50 grams parmesan cheese

salt and pepper

SAUCE

100ml cream

80 grams strong Blue King Island Roaring Forties Blue

Heat the oven to 180°C.

To prepare the tomatoes slice the top of each tomato, leave the green stalk on for presentation if you like. Scoop out the seeds and pulp and set aside.

Crush the garlic, finely dice the onion and sauté them in a heavy based pan with the extra virgin olive oil and butter until soft. Add the tomato seeds and pulp, cook over a low heat to reduce the liquid away. Toss through the herbs and lentils and season well with salt and pepper.

Fill each tomato with the filling and place the lid back on top. Put the tomatoes into a baking dish and drizzle with the extra virgin olive oil and bake for around 15 minutes until the tomato is cooked and the filling is heated through, but the tomatoes are not overcooked and soggy.

To make the polenta, finely dice the onion, crush the garlic and sauté them in a small pot with the butter. Slice the mushrooms and add them to the pot and cook until they are soft. Add the milk to the pot and bring it to a simmer. Add the polenta to the pot, stirring well until the polenta is soft and cooked - it should not feel grainy when rubbed between your fingers. Add the grated cheese and season well with salt and pepper.

To make the sauce simply heat the cream and chopped cheeses, stirring well until smooth.

Serve immediately.

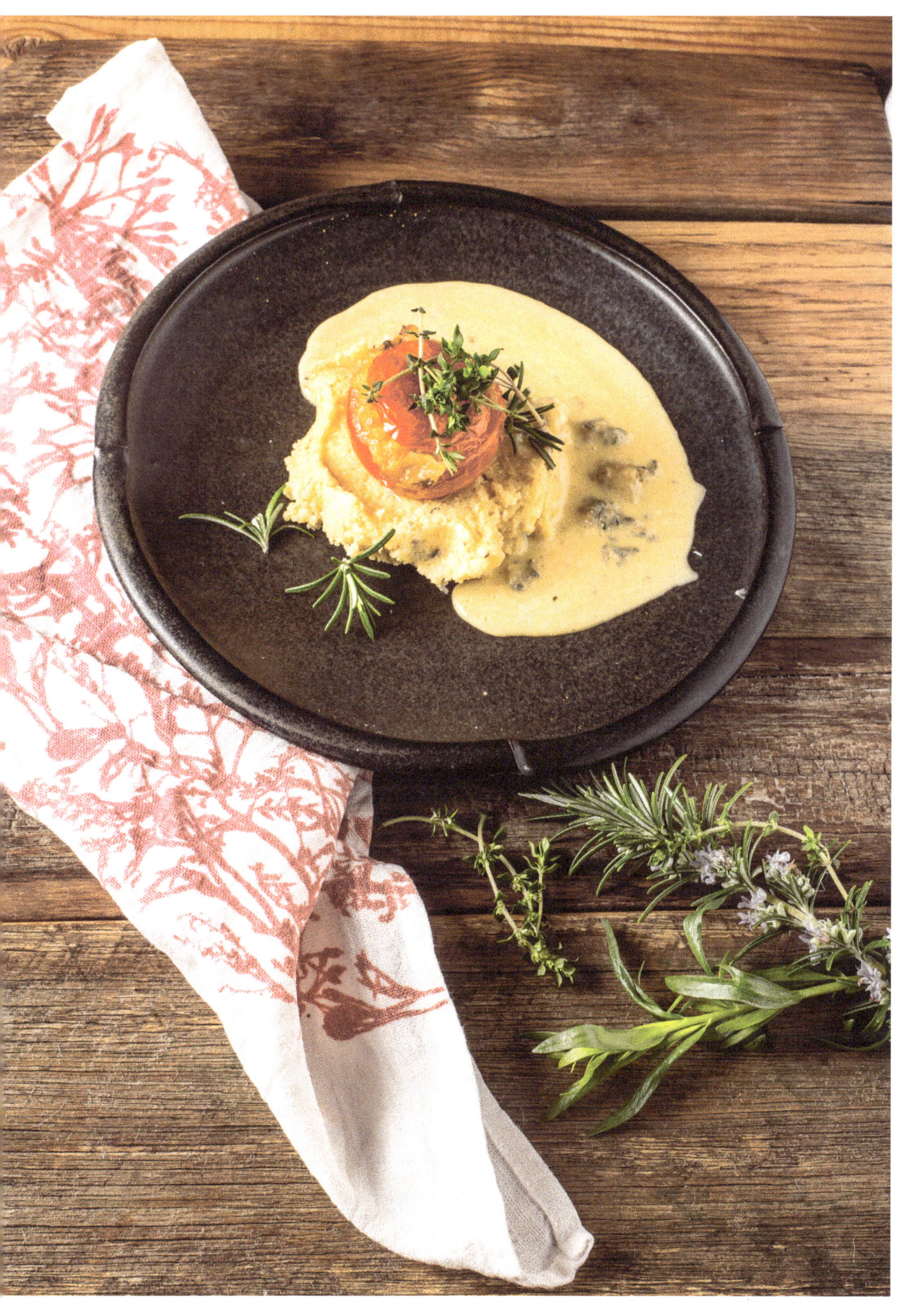

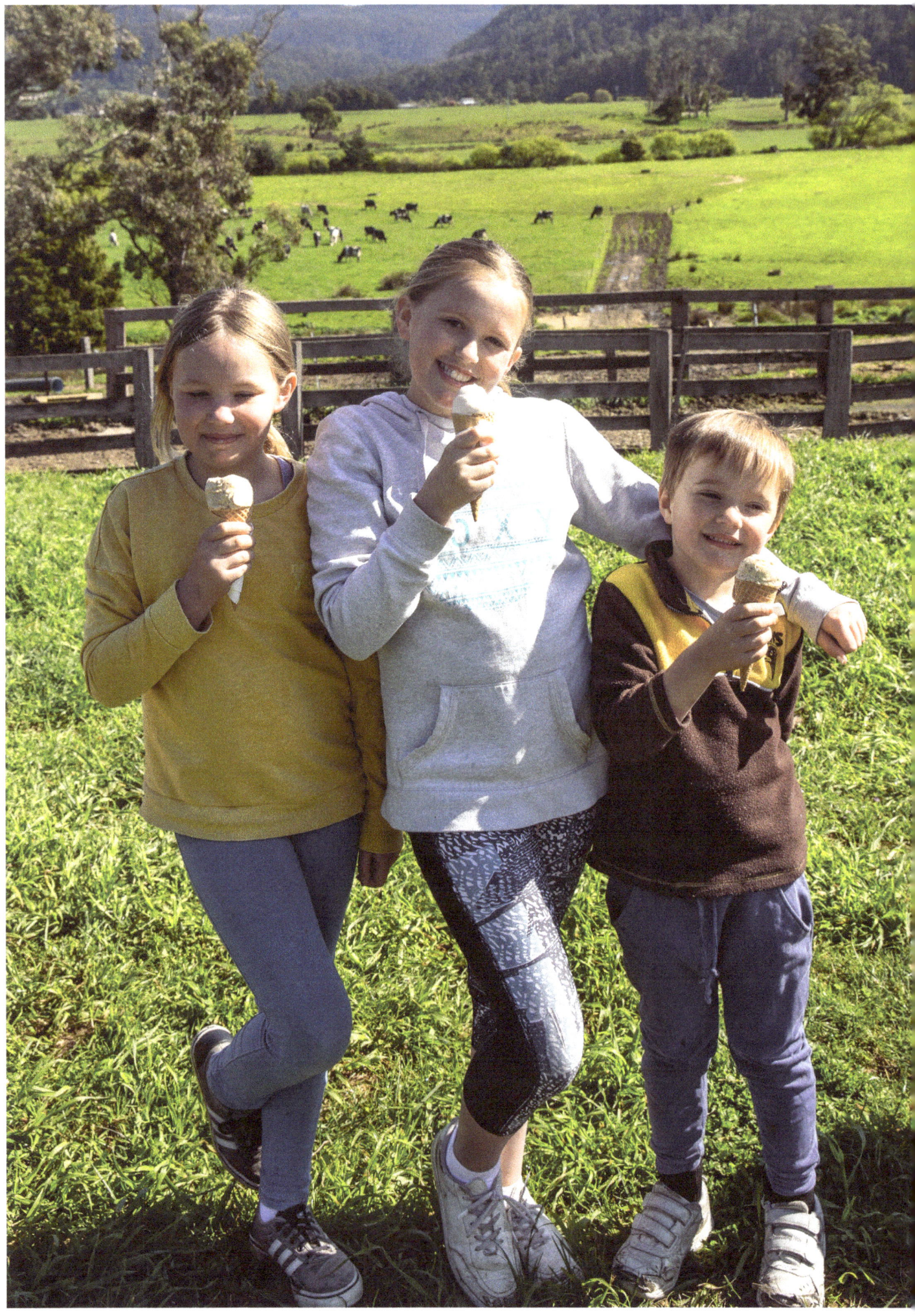

"If my family is eating five veg and a few fruits a day I am not too bothered by what else.
If the veggies are not getting eaten then I need to look at and re-assess what they are filling up on."

Wallaby Shanks Braised with Paprika

SERVES 6 OR MORE

12 wallaby shanks

3 tablespoons flour

2 large onions

6 cloves garlic

2 tablespoons robust extra virgin olive oil

4 bay leaves

4 sprigs thyme

2 carrots

2 sticks celery

1 leek

600 grams tomato

400ml beef stock (at least - may need more to cover depending on your dish)

1 tablespoon paprika. I use Weston Farm Smoked Paprika

sea salt

cracked pepper

TO SERVE

Polenta (see page 78 for recipe) try swapping the mushrooms for cauliflower or pumpkin!

Heat the oven to 160°C.

Cover the shanks in flour by popping the shanks and flour into a bag and give them a good shake. Heat a large pan with the olive oil, seal and brown the wallaby shanks on all sides.

Lay the shanks into a baking dish with a lid. Peel and dice the onion, celery, carrot and leek and crush the garlic, add them to the baking dish with the bay leaves, thyme, tomato, stock and paprika. Cover with baking paper and then kitchen foil if you don't have a lid for your baking dish.

Cook for 2-3 hours until the meat is tender and falling from the bone. Season with salt and pepper.

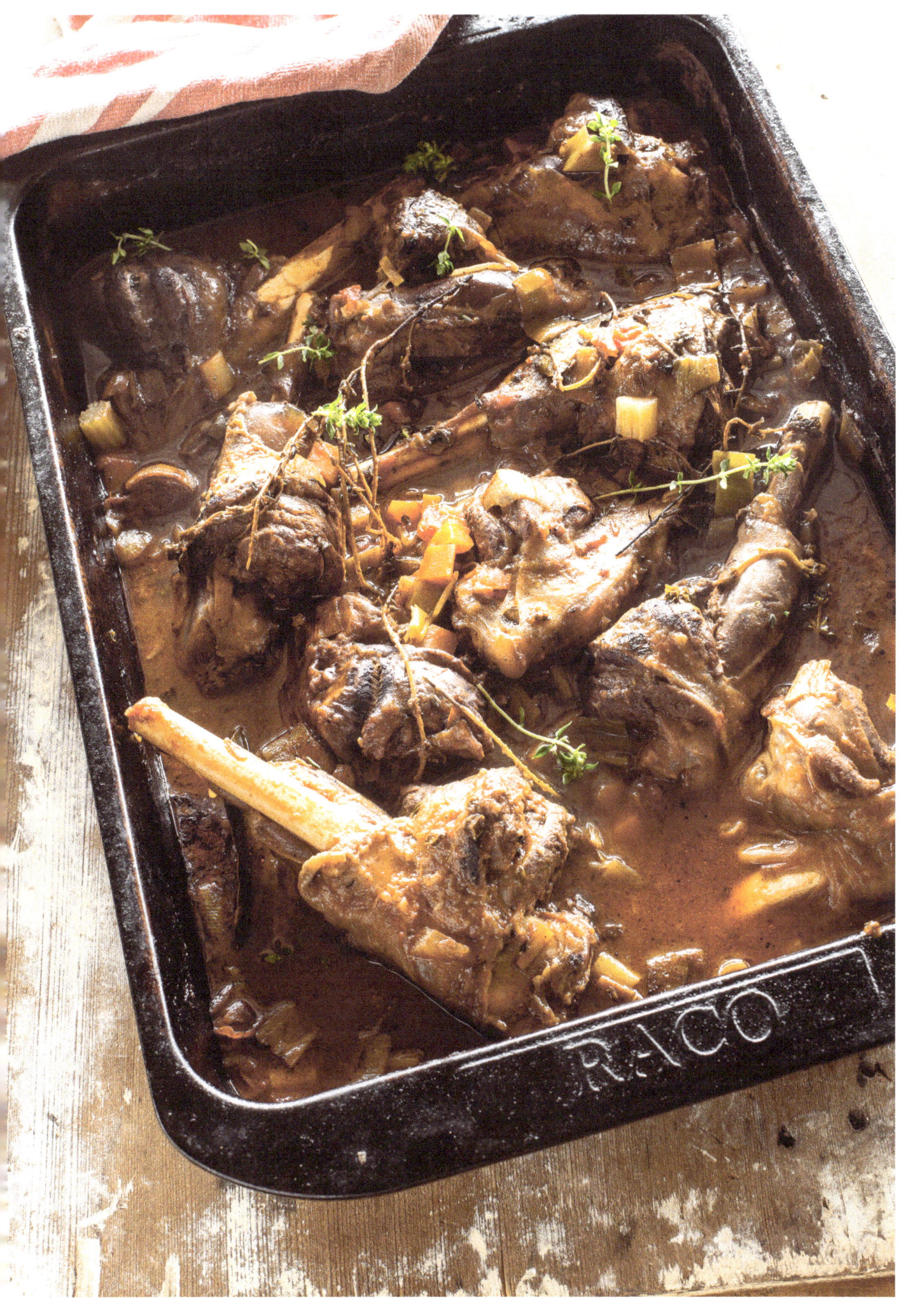

Octopus Baked with Tomato, Olives and Jalapenos

SERVES 6

Serve this octopus with cooked pasta or crusty bread and salad.

1 kilo octopus

2 onions

4 cloves garlic

2 bay leaves

2 sprigs thyme

2 sprigs oregano

2 tablespoons Weston Farm smoked paprika

2 tablespoons basil

cracked pepper

sea salt

800 grams tomato

60 grams kalamata olives

jalapeno peppers or hot chillies (or add pickled jalapenos to finish)

extra virgin olive oil

TO SERVE

marinated feta and cooked pasta or crusty bread and salad

Heat the oven to 160°C.

Clean the octopus by pulling all the skin off the tentacle. Peel and slice the onion and peel and crush the garlic. Lay the garlic and the onions and the octopus into a heavy based baking dish. Add the bay leaves, thyme, oregano, pepper, sea salt, olive oil and tomato.

Cover with baking paper and kitchen foil and bake for 2 hours or until tender. Toss through the jalapeno pepper and pitted olives and top with feta.

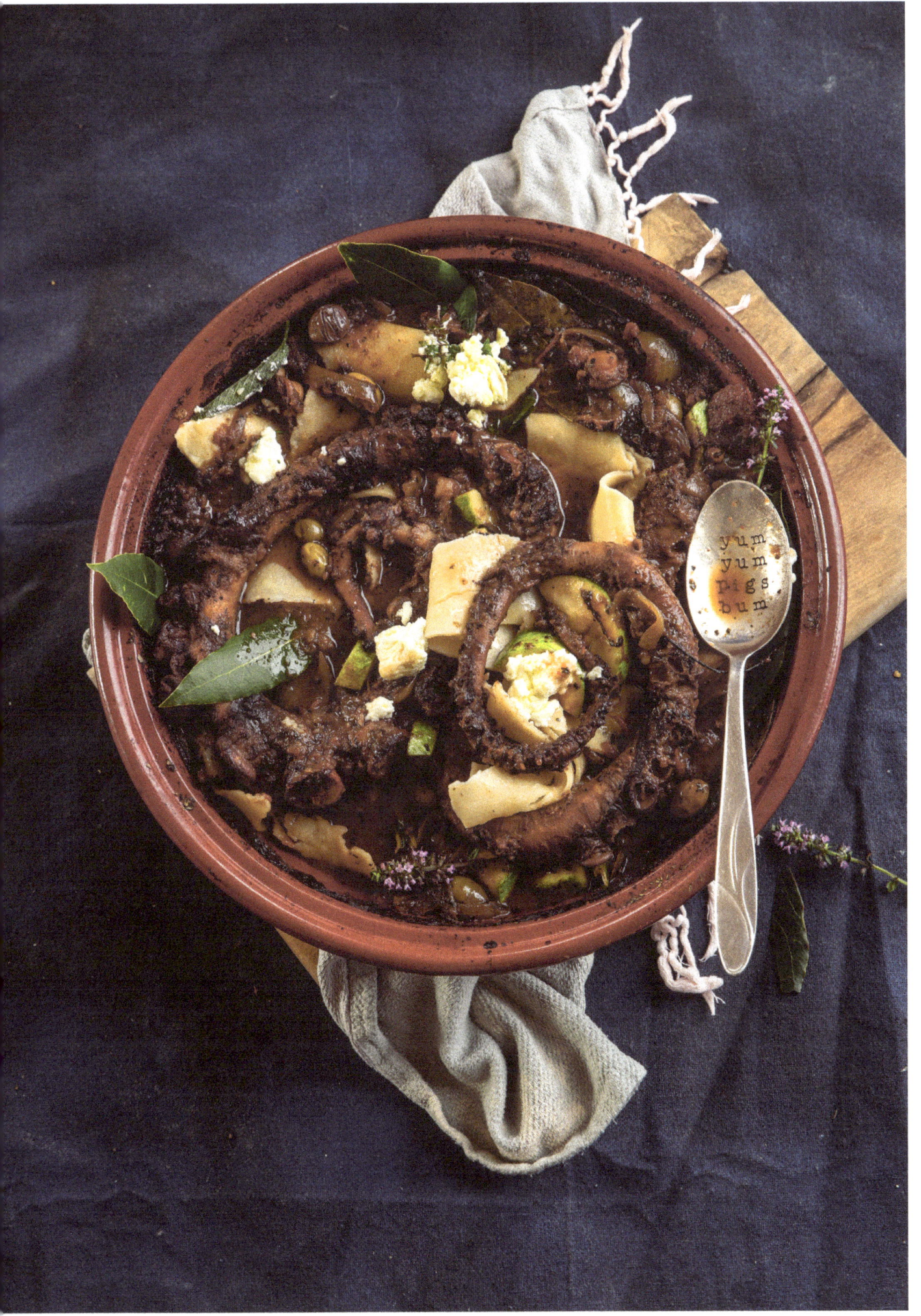

BREAM CREEK VINEYARD

Pork Belly, Apple and Fennel cooked in Bream Creek Vineyard Sauvignon Blanc

SERVES 6

It is hard to beat the belly of the pork for a tasty and tender cut. Remove the skin if you want to prepare it for crackle as this is slow cooked it won't crackle well. To achieve a nice crackle, cover the skin in salt and rub in well, leave for an hour. Heat the oven as hot as you can and rub fresh salt and oil into the skin, place the skin on a tray and bake for about 20 minutes.

1 large piece of pork belly - about 1 kilo

2 onions

4 apples (or apple paste or preserved)

1 large fennel bulb

6 cloves garlic

3 bay leaves

6 sprigs thyme

10 peppercorns

300ml Bream Creek Vineyard Sauvignon Blanc

1 litre stock (beef, veg, chicken)

TO SERVE

apple slaw or mashed potatoes, or polenta and vegetables

Heat the oven to 160°C.

Seal the piece of pork in a large pan over a medium high heat so it is browned all over, lay the pork in a baking dish or you could use your slow cooker (adjust the cooking time).

Peel and slice the onion, slice the fennel, remove the core form the apples and chop into pieces, peel the garlic and add to the dish. Add the whole cloves of garlic, bay leaves, thyme, peppercorns and cover with the wine and stock.

Cover with kitchen foil and bake for 1.5-3 hours until cooked through. Size, thickness, amount of fat is all going to affect the cooking time, its best to put on early or even the day before. To tell if it is cooked you should be able to poke it with a spoon and the meat will fall apart.

Purée the cooking liquid and apples to create a delicious sauce.

Serve with mashed potato or a tasty slaw such as an apple cider dressed apple, cabbage and carrot slaw.

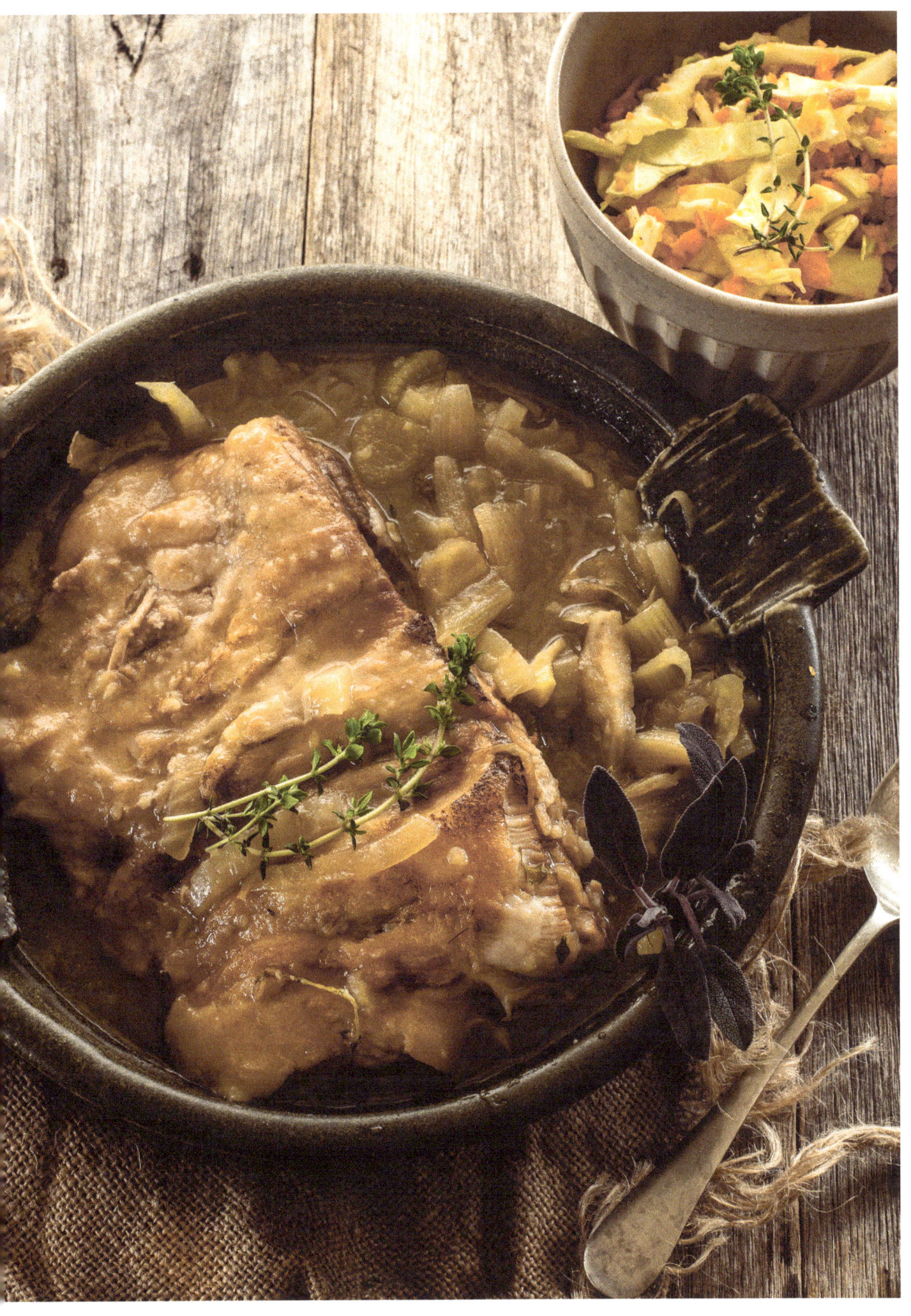

Leek and Apple Soup with Freshfield Grove Lemon Agrumato

SERVES 4

An agrumato extra virgin olive oil is produced by adding the flavour/fruit to the press when pressing the oil resulting in an authentic flavour. Not an infusion, generally the flavour is a lot more punchy and prominent in the oil. For this recipe use fresh apples or apples you have bottled or frozen. Yes, I bottle apples, it may seem odd but my freezers are full of bones, octopus, leeks, crushed garlic, stocks and seafood so I avoid freezing my fruit when I can get away with it.

1 tablespoon extra virgin olive oil

3 leeks

3 cloves garlic

1 onion

1 kilo apples

1 litre veg or chicken stock

3 sprigs tarragon

1 teaspoon fennel seed

salt

white pepper

200ml cream

60ml lemon Freshfield Grove agrumato

In a large heavy based pot heat the oil, add the roughly chopped leek that has been split in halves lengthways and washed. Peel and roughly chop the garlic and onion, add to the pan and sauté until soft and coloured.

Add the apples that have had the cores removed, stock, fennel seed and tarragon and simmer until the apples and leeks are soft and cooked through.

Purée and season with salt and pepper add the cream and heat through and serve with a drizzle of the agrumato oil.

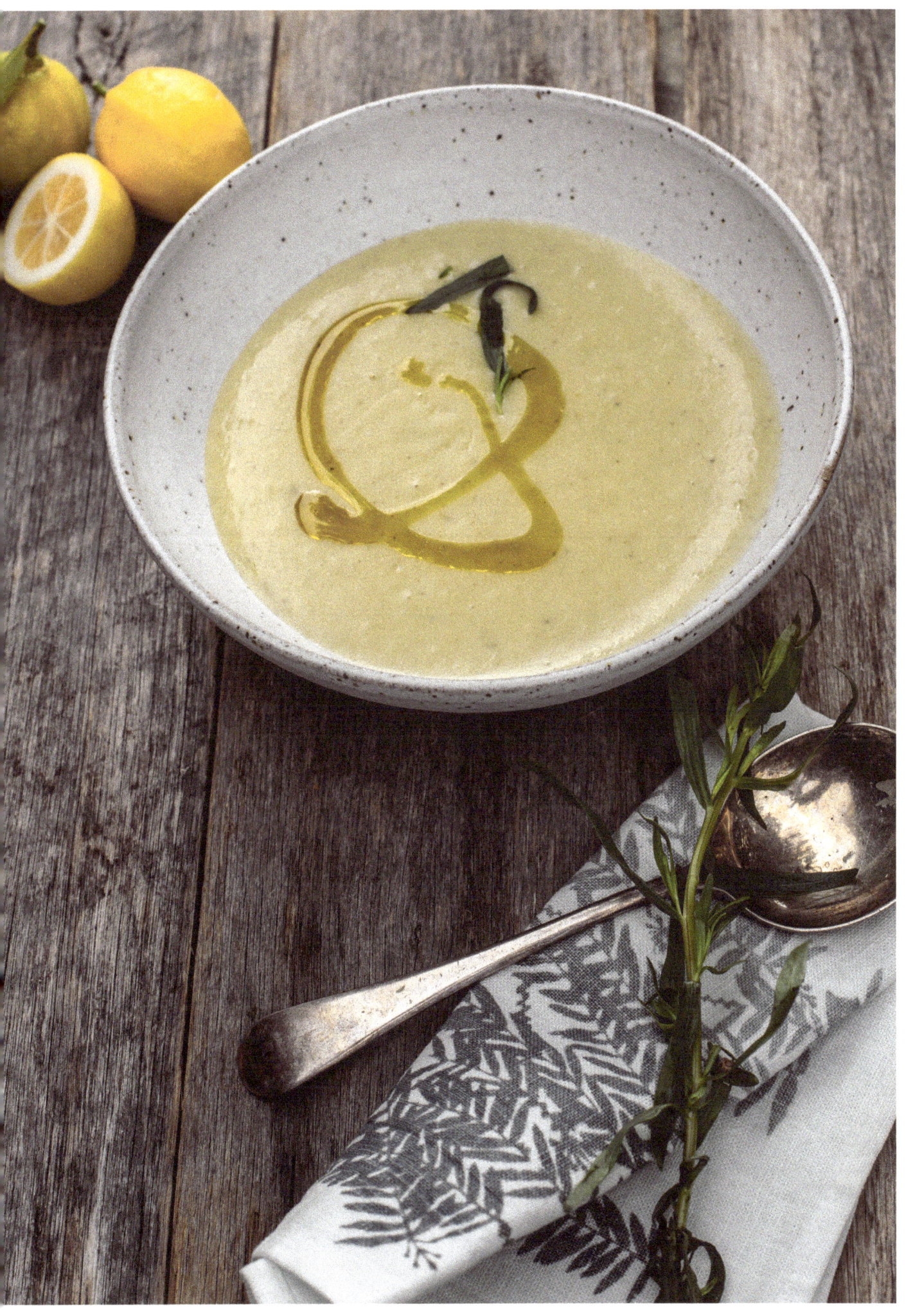

Oysters with Lemon Agrumato and Pickled Fennel

MAKES 1 DOZEN

I find most people who love oysters love to eat them simply natural with maybe some lemon. So, when I serve them I like to have platters of natural oysters with maybe an interesting topping that people can add if they wish or simply choose to devour the oyster natural. This sweet and spicy pickle is a perfect complement to the salty fresh oyster.

1 dozen Cameron of Tasmania pacific oysters

1 cup vinegar

1 cup sugar

fennel bulb and fronds

1 small red chilli

Freshfield Grove lemon agrumato

Finely dice the fennel and crush the chilli. In a pot bring the sugar and vinegar to the boil. Add the fennel and leave at least overnight but this will store in the refrigerator for a few weeks also delicious with a fish burger.

Shuck the oysters and top with the pickle and a good dash of lemon agrumato.

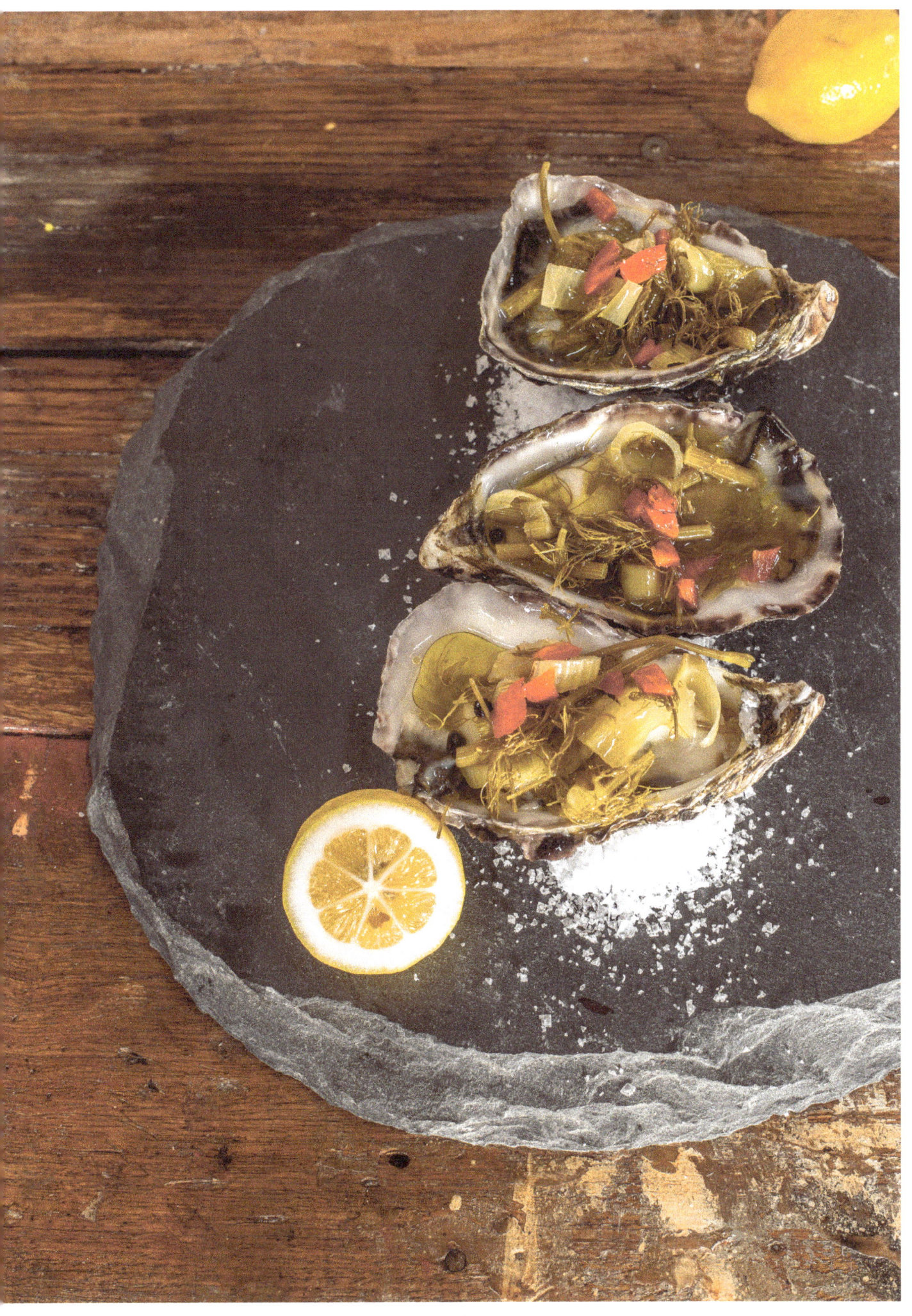

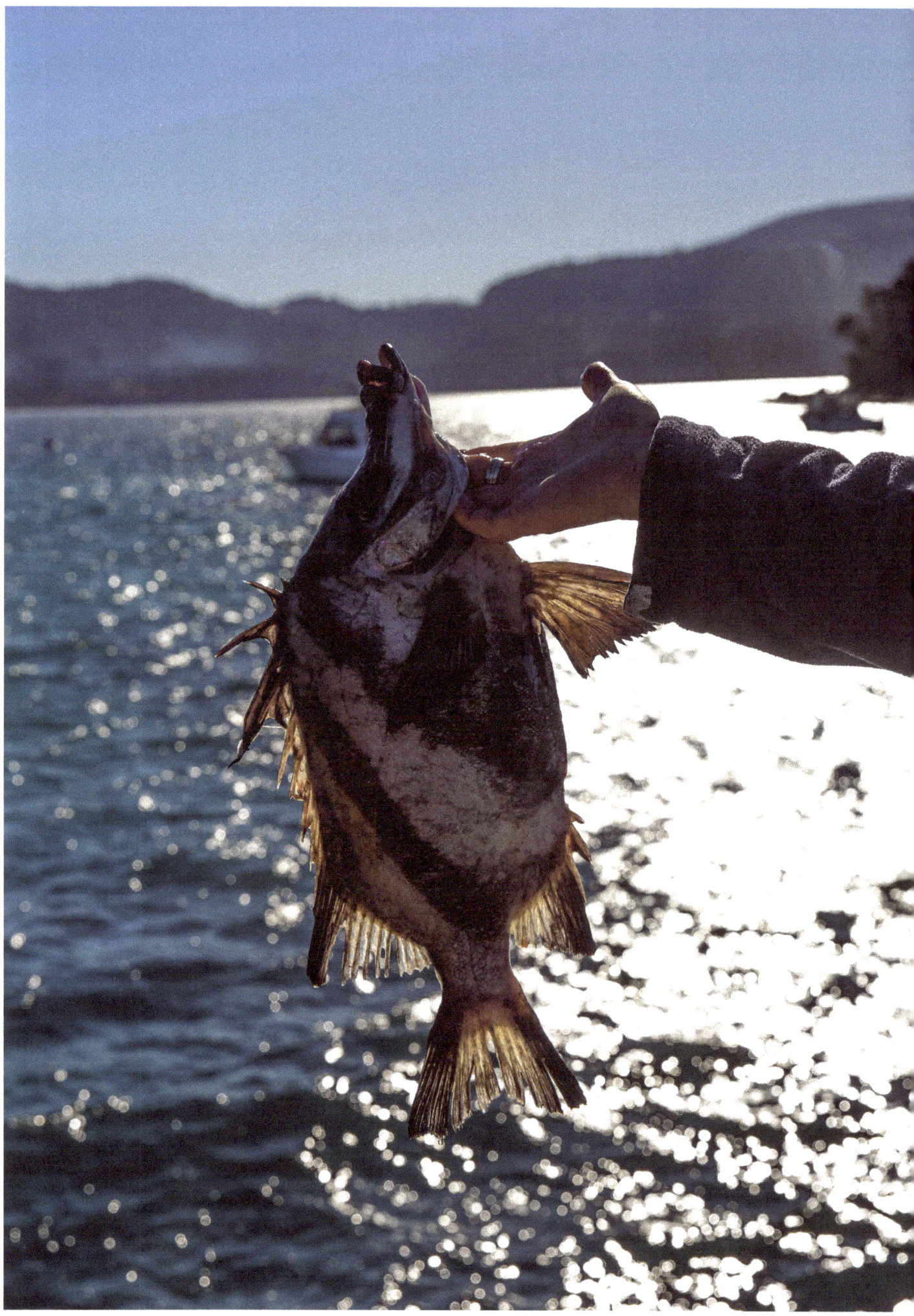

"We may think a high quality well produced ingredient is expensive, but compared to takeaway, it is not at all."

Duck Confit served with Puddleduck Vineyard Pinot Noir Jam and Slaw

SERVES 6

Duck confit is a classic, delicious and beautiful dish to prepare for an almost impossible to muck up impressive dinner party dish. Traditionally, to confit the duck, it is cooked in its own fat, but a full flavoured robust extra virgin olive oil will add plenty of flavour (not to mention not add any more saturated fat to the dish!). The duck confit is gorgeous served on top of a risotto such as mushroom and gruyere or with a mash potato or parsnip. I have served it here with a slaw, as I find it is good to have some crisp veggies and apple to break up the delicious fat. Maryland is the cut of poultry that is the leg and thigh together.

6 duck marylands

extra virgin olive oil

SLAW

1 tablespoon apple cider vinegar

2 tablespoons robust extra virgin olive oil

1 green apple

⅛ red cabbage

2 carrots

3 spring onion

sea salt

white pepper

PINOT NOIR JAM

300ml Puddleduck Vineyard Pinot Noir

2 red onions

3 tablespoons brown sugar

Heat the oven to 160°C

In a large heavy based pan seal the duck maryland's making sure the skin sides gets an extra minute for a crispy skin. Place the maryland in a baking dish. The trick here is to find a dish where they fit snuggly into when laid out flat - so you won't need as much oil to cover them.

Cover the marylands with oil then cover the dish with foil and cook in a 120°C oven for around 4 hours until the meat is tender and falling from the bone. The leftover oil can be stored in the fridge to use in the next few days for your cooking.

To make the slaw, finely slice or grate the apple, carrot, spring onion and mix with the vinegar and oil, season well with the salt and pepper.

To make the jam, finely slice the red onion and sauté in a heavy based pan with the oil, add the brown sugar and wine and continue to cook until the jam reduces into a thick sauce this will take around 30 minutes on a low heat.

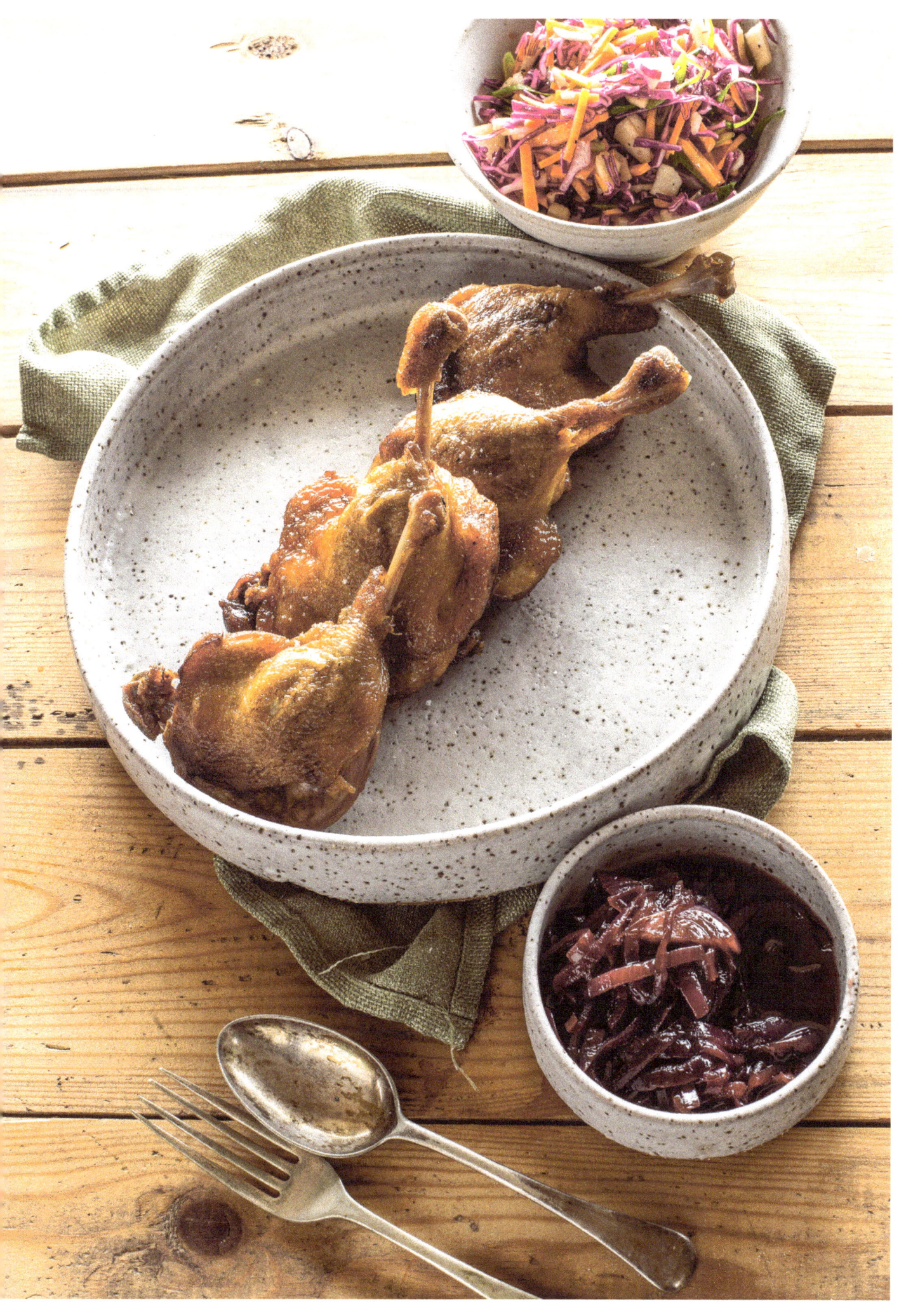

Recipe by Maggie Emmett

Goats Cheese Ravioli with Brown Butter and Sage

SERVES 2-4

PASTA

180 grams plain flour

2 large eggs

FILLING

100 grams goats cheese - my favourite is Tongola Curdy

1 egg for egg wash

SAUCE

1 tablespoon butter

extra virgin olive oil

3 cloves garlic

40 sage leaves

sea salt

cracked pepper

TO SERVE

a big salad

To make the pasta, either in the food processor or a bowl mix the egg into the flour and knead well. Starting with the widest opening on the pasta machine roll the dough out through the pasta machine, decreasing opening each time until you have thin sheets of pasta, but not to thin, this is number 5 on our pasta making machine.

Put a large pot of water on to boil. On a very well floured bench lay the pasta sheets. Place tablespoons of goats cheese down one side of the sheet length ways about 8cm apart, egg wash around the cheese and fold the sheet of pasta over to create a fat pillow of cheese. Work quick here to get the ravioli into the pot promptly, if it sits around on the bench the cheese will start to soggy the pasta and it will all stick to the bench.

Cook the ravioli for about 3 minutes in boiling water.

While the pasta is cooking quickly heat the pan with the extra virgin olive oil and the butter and then when it froths and just starts to go brown toss through the garlic and sage leaves and a big pinch of sea salt and pepper, toss through the pasta and serve.

If you wanted to prep the ravioli the day before then cook and cool it in ice water, drain and refrigerate it rolled in a little oil if you need. Then simply dunk the ravioli back in the boiling water to serve.

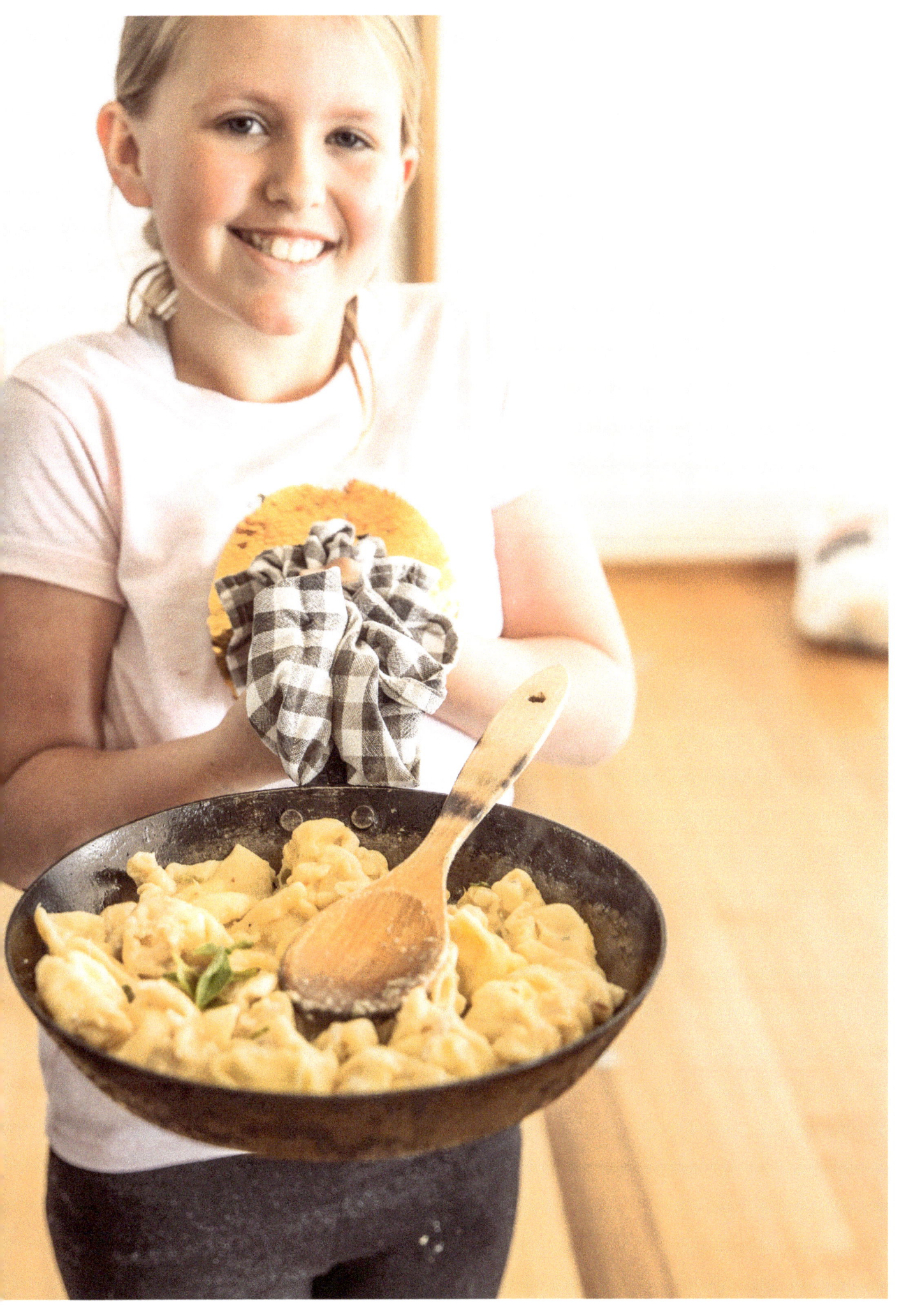

Scallops and Handmade Pasta

SERVES 4

300 grams fresh pasta
(to make your own see page 96)

1 large brown onion

3 cloves garlic

1 large red chilli

400 grams scallop meat

2 tablespoons tarragon

sea salt

cracked pepper

2 tablespoons extra virgin olive oil

80 grams parmesan

To cook the pasta, bring a large pot of boiling water to the boil. The pasta will only take a few minutes to cook so be ready to cook it when you start cooking the scallops.

To cook the scallops, in a large heavy based pan over a medium high heat, heat the olive oil and sauté the peeled and finely sliced onion, crushed garlic and chilli stirring often until soft and cooked.

Make sure the pan is still at a high heat and add the scallops, do not overcrowd the pan or stew the scallops. The scallops will only need a few minutes to cook turned once or twice, until cooked through, then toss through the hot cooked pasta and serve topped with the cheese.

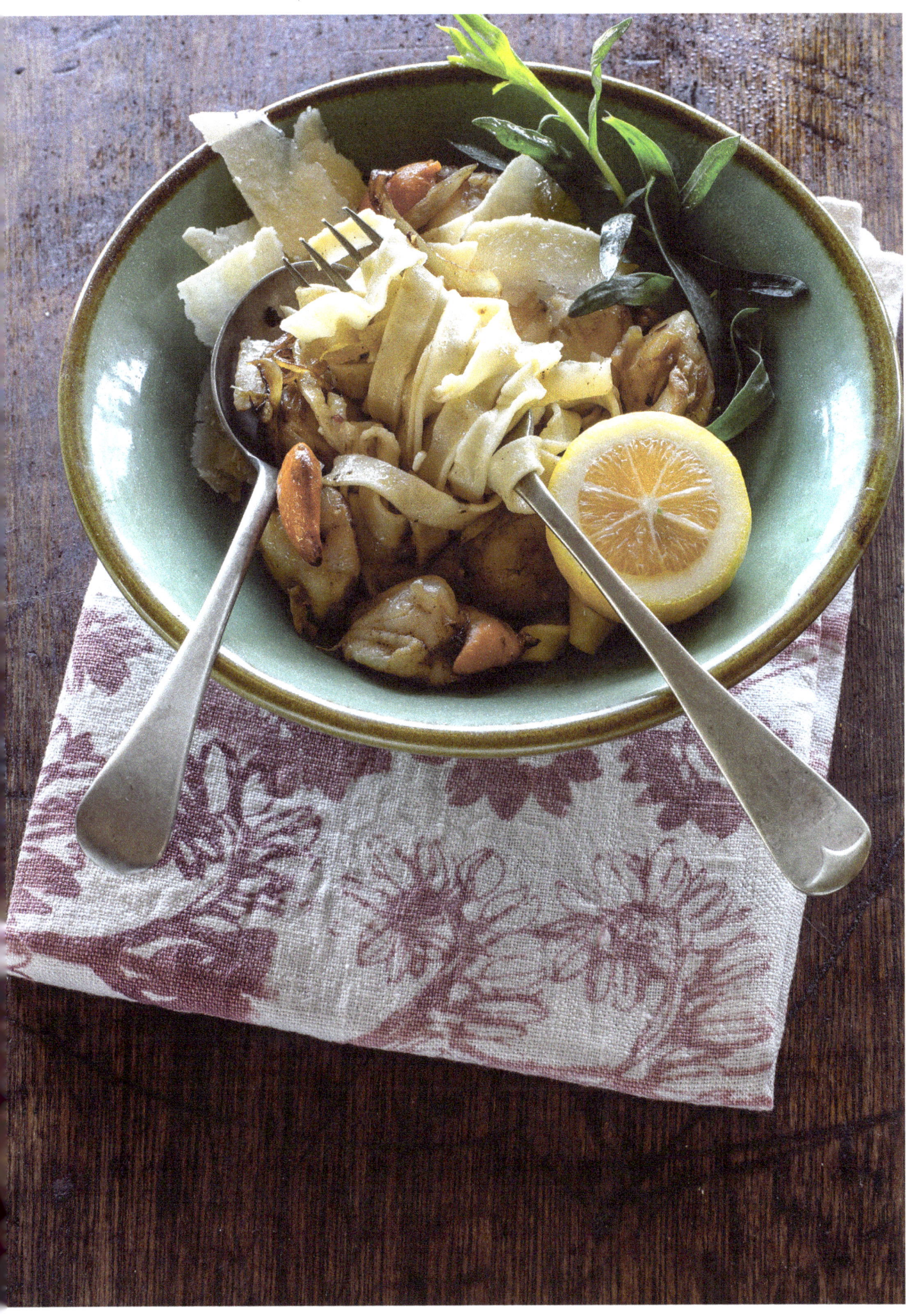

Beer Battered Scallops with Tartare Sauce

SERVE 4-6

I thought I didn't like deep fried food until I started deep-frying with extra virgin olive oil. It was that stench and taste of bad oil I did not like. Extra virgin olive oil doesn't make you feel 'greasy' after you've eaten it, and has a fresh flavour. It can handle up to 6 hours of cooking before it loses its nutritional values. After I have used it in my deep fryer, I strain and store the oil in the fridge and use it up quickly in other cooking such as pan frying fish or baking octopus. Filling your little deep fryer up with extra virgin olive oil is worth it at least once a year for fresh scallops.

500 grams scallop meat

1 cup flour

1 ½ cups self raising flour

375ml can Cascade beer

1 tablespoon vinegar

sea salt

extra virgin olive oil for frying

TARTARE

1 tablespoon white vinegar

1 tablespoon dill

1 egg yolk

approximately 100ml extra virgin olive oil

1 tablespoon capers

1 tablespoon gherkins

pepper

TO SERVE

a big salad

To make the tartare, crack the egg into the blender add the white vinegar and begin blending, drizzle the oil in a thin stream to create a thick mayonnaise. Add the chopped capers, gherkins and dill and season with pepper.

To make the batter whisk the self raising flour and the beer together to create a smooth batter. Heat the oil in a heavy based pan or wok, about 2cm deep to 170°C or fill the deep fryer. Roll the scallops in the flour and then dip each scallop into the batter and carefully drop into the oil until golden brown and the scallop is cooked through.

Remove from the oil and drain on paper before serving hot and sprinkled with sea salt, the tartare sauce and a big salad.

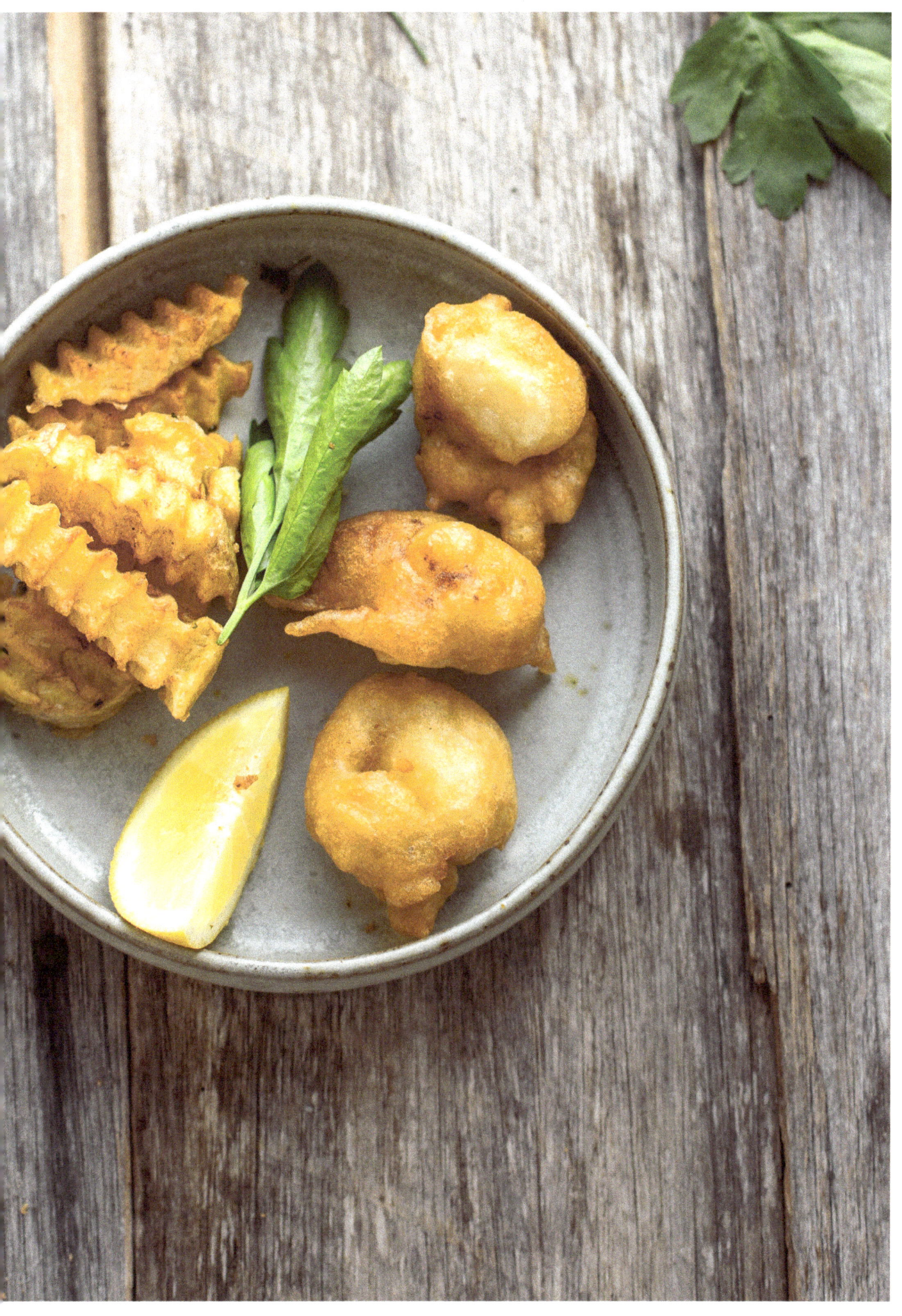

TASFOODS LTD, MEANDER VALLEY DAIRY

Meander Valley Dairy Scones

SERVES 10-12

These scones are so easy to pull together in a short time. Pair with finger sandwiches and hot tea to create an authentic High Tea.

2 cups self raising flour, plus extra for dusting

2 teaspoons baking powder

2 teaspoons salt

1 egg

50 grams cold Meander Valley Dairy unsalted cultured butter, diced

125ml Meander Valley Dairy Traditional Buttermilk, plus extra for wash

raspberry jam and Meander Valley Double Cream to serve

Heat the oven to 200°C. Line a baking tray.

Sift flour, baking powder and salt together in a large mixing bowl. Rub the butter into the flour with your fingertips until it resembles breadcrumbs. Alternatively, pulse the mixture in a food processor until you get the same result.

Create a well in the middle of the flour mixture. Whisk together buttermilk and eggs, pour into the well. Cut the flour with a knife to blend the milk into the flour until it comes together.

Turn the dough onto a floured bench top and lightly bring the dough together (it is important to handle the dough as little as possible so it stays light). Pat out into a 2.5cm thickness. Using a round cutter, cut the dough into portions. Place the scones onto the lined baking tray and lightly brush with milk.

Bake for 12 minutes until golden and brown. Serve with raspberry jam and a dollop of double cream.

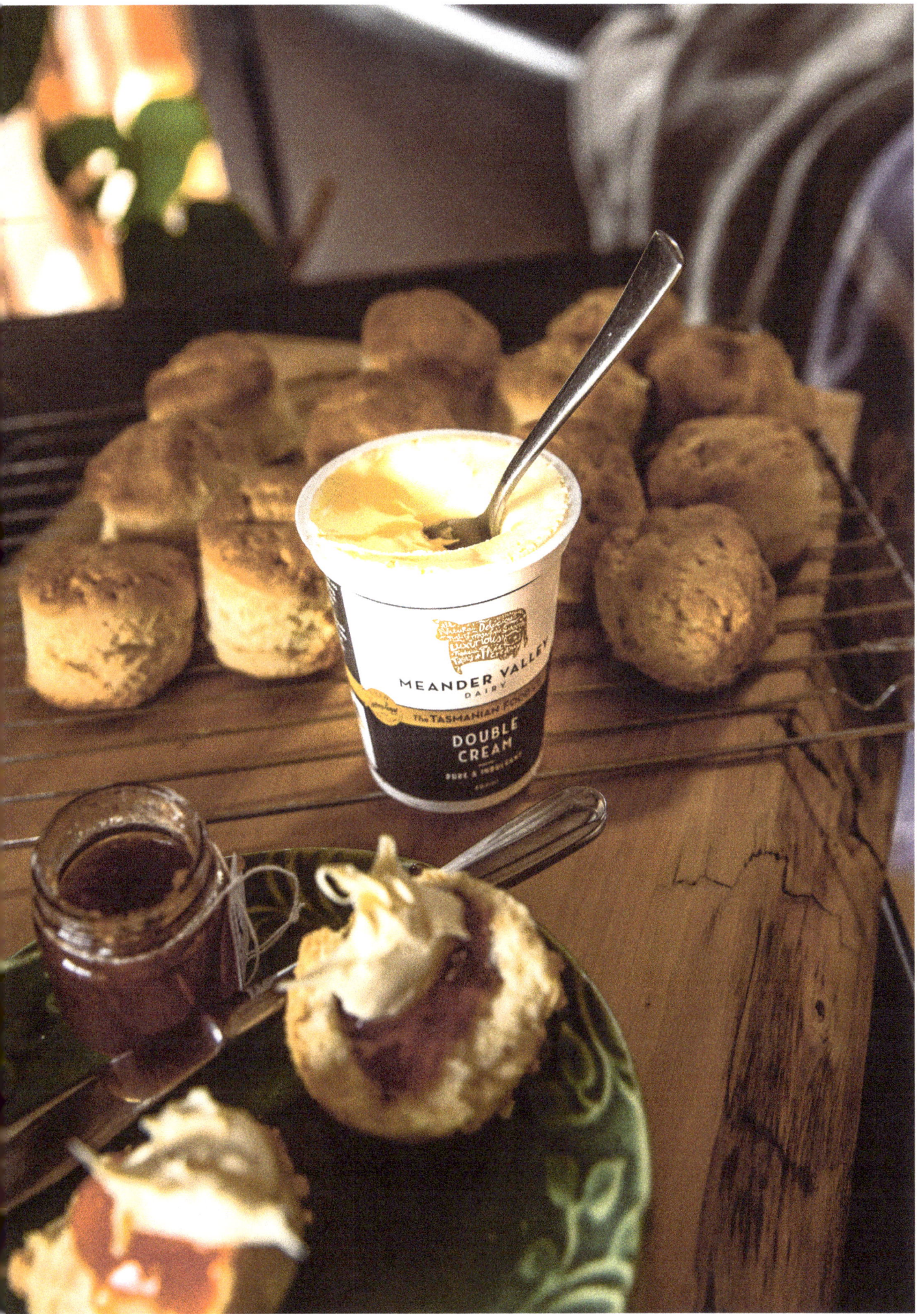

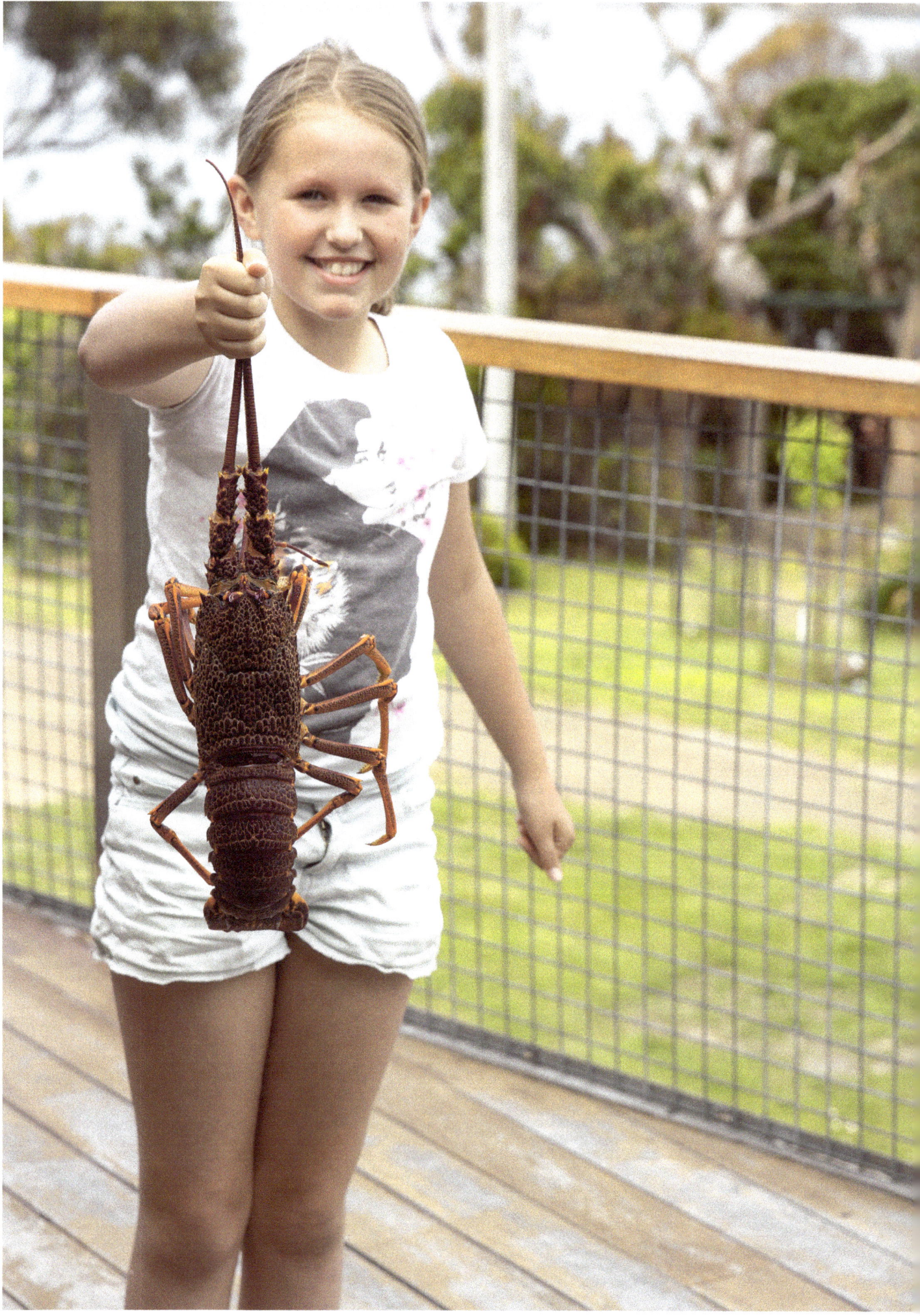

"Yes, having children in the kitchen may send you a little cray cray, but persevere... having a meal cooked for you by your own child is priceless."

Garlic and Herb Pull Apart

MAKES 1 LOAF

I've won first prize at the Bream Creek Show Hall of Industries for quite a few years in a row with this recipe. This beautiful bread can turn a simple soup lunch into something special.

BREAD DOUGH

500 grams plain or bakers flour

1 teaspoon yeast

1 teaspoon salt

1 teaspoon sugar

1 teaspoon bread improver

300ml - 320ml luke warm water

FOR THE GARLIC BUTTER

4 cloves garlic

½ bunch fresh parsley

1 tablespoon fresh basil

1 tablespoon fresh oregano

1 tablespoon rosemary

1 tablespoon extra virgin olive oil

½ teaspoon sea salt

¼ teaspoon cracked pepper

To make the herb and garlic butter whip all ingredients together in the blender.

Knead all the bread ingredients together to create a smooth dough. I do this in the thermocooker with the knead function for 2 minutes. Alternatively mix by hand in a bowl and knead for around 10 minutes on a floured bench.

Place the dough in a bowl and cover and leave dough to rise in a warm spot for 30 minutes or until doubled in size.

Heat the oven to 180°C.

Roll onto a floured board into large rectangle and spread herb butter over dough.

If necessary, sprinkle dough with flour first to prevent butter from sliding off.

With a butter knife, cut 3-4cm wide strips. Fold each dough strip in half lengthways and place cut side up in a 26cm spring form tin until all the strips are pressed in together. Leave to rise in a warm spot for about 20 minutes until it is filling the tin well. Bake for approximately 40-45 minutes. Serve hot.

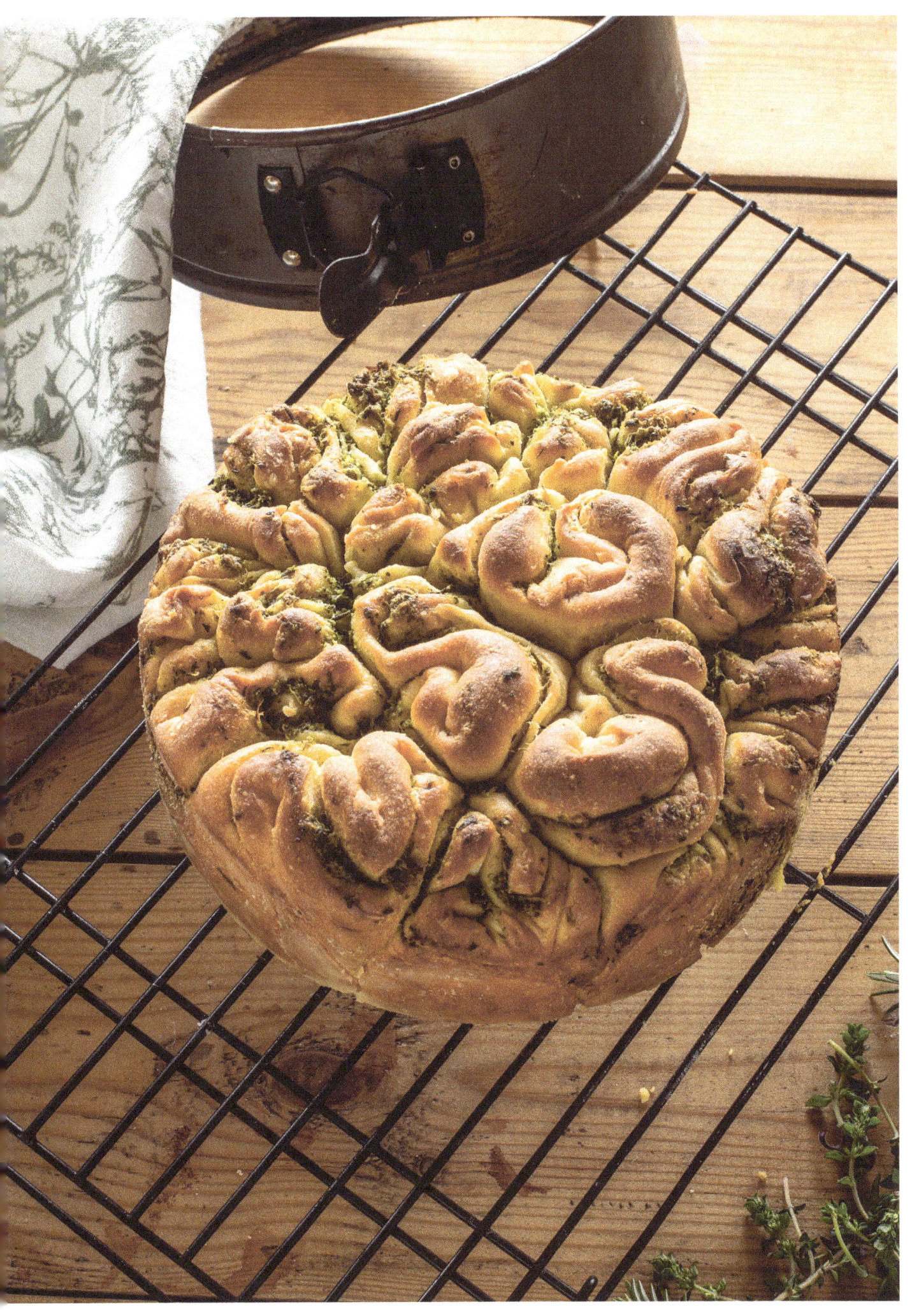

Garlic, Feta and Herb Pizza

MAKES 2 LARGE PIZZAS

Use this simple base for the base of 2 large pizzas I love baking bread and I love making my own pizzas for the family. My kids can choose the toppings and I know exactly what we are eating.

500 grams flour

1 teaspoon yeast

1 teaspoon salt

1 teaspoon sugar

300ml - 320ml water

robust extra virgin olive oil

sea salt

2 tablespoons garlic

100 grams feta

4 tablespoons aromatic herbs such as rosemary, basil oregano, parsley

sea salt

Heat the oven to 200°C.

To make the dough knead all ingredients well, I use the thermocooker or you can use any mixer or knead by hand on the bench for around 10 minutes to produce a smooth firm dough.

Cover and leave to rise in a warm position until the dough has doubled in size. Knock the dough back down and divide into 2 and roll into tight balls.

Roll the dough out into large (around 30cm diameter) pizza bases and lay the bases on a baking tray rubbed with some of the extra virgin olive oil, and then sprinkle on the finely chopped herbs, crushed garlic and feta and drizzle with the oil and a sprinkle of sea salt.

If you like a thin base be ready to cook your pizza straightaway. If you like it thicker leave it to rise after you have put your toppings on.

Bake for around 15-20 minutes or until golden brown and cooked through.

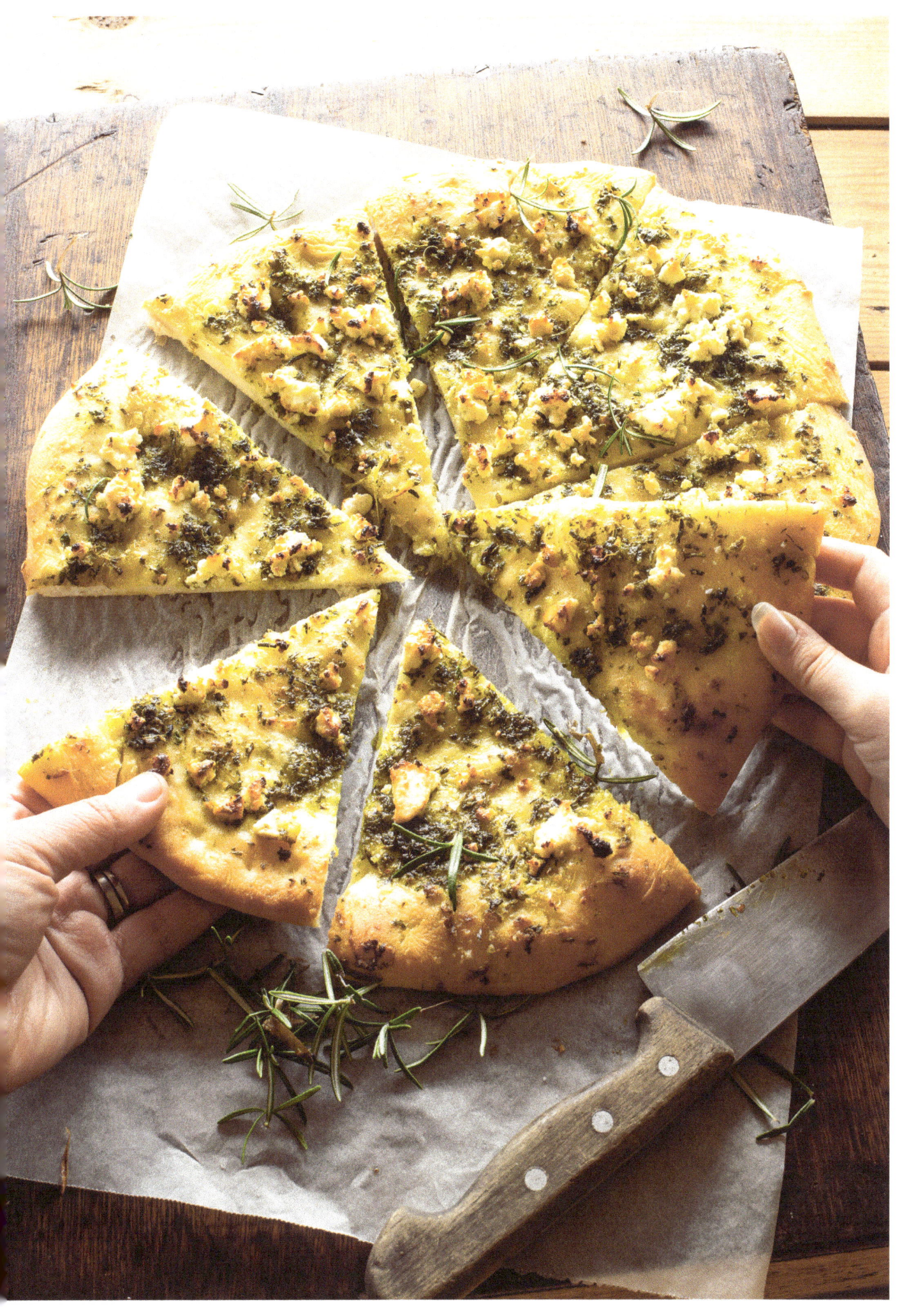

Apple Cinnamon and Honey Porridge

SERVES 6

This can be baked with chunks of whole seasonal fruits for a delicious easy to serve breakfast. Use frozen or preserved fruits.

400ml milk

180ml water

2 apples

180 grams oats

1 tablespoon honey

1 teaspoon cinnamon

Place grated apple and all ingredients in a heavy based saucepan. Bring to a gentle boil and simmer stirring regularly for about 8 minutes. Cover and rest for about 10 minutes to thicken and serve.

Or in your thermocooker, quarter the apples and put in the mixing bowl, grate, speed 6 for 3 seconds. Add all other ingredients cook at 12 minutes/90°C speed 2/ reverse. Leave to rest for 10 minutes covered to finish cooking before serving.

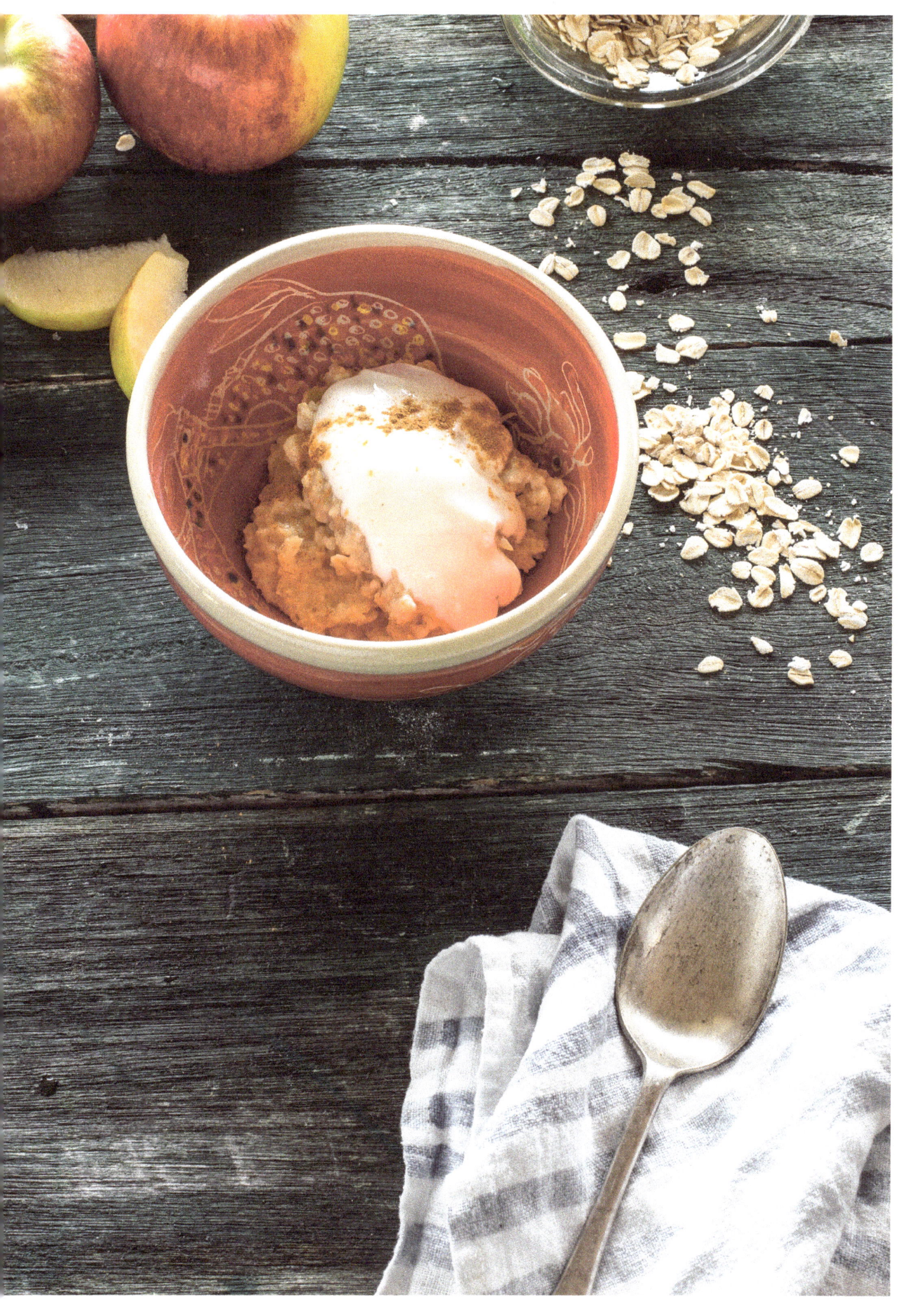

Overnight Oat Ideas

SERVES 4-6 FOR BREAKFAST OR SNACKS

We find overnight oats to be a simple breakfast prepared earlier for a quick nutritious breakfast on a busy morning. Use whatever seasonal fresh fruits you can access or persevered, frozen or canned fruits when not in season.

APPLE, RASPBERRY AND LAVENDER

I am lucky to have apple trees that produce a good amount of fruit but finding ways to use all my preserved fruit, without making endless dessert can be a challenge, so I make this breakfast regularly.

2 apples (fresh grated, stewed frozen or bottled)

½ cup raspberries, fresh or frozen

1 cup oats

1 cup milk

1 teaspoon culinary lavender

100ml yogurt

Mix together and leave overnight in the refrigerator.

PEANUT BUTTER

3 tablespoons Old Spikey Bridge peanut butter

1 cup oats

⅛ cup yogurt

1 tablespoon honey

1 cup milk

Mix together and leave overnight in the refrigerator.

QUINCE AND MIXED BERRY

½ cup berries

½ cup preserved quince

1 cup oats

1 cup milk

Mix together and leave overnight in the refrigerator.

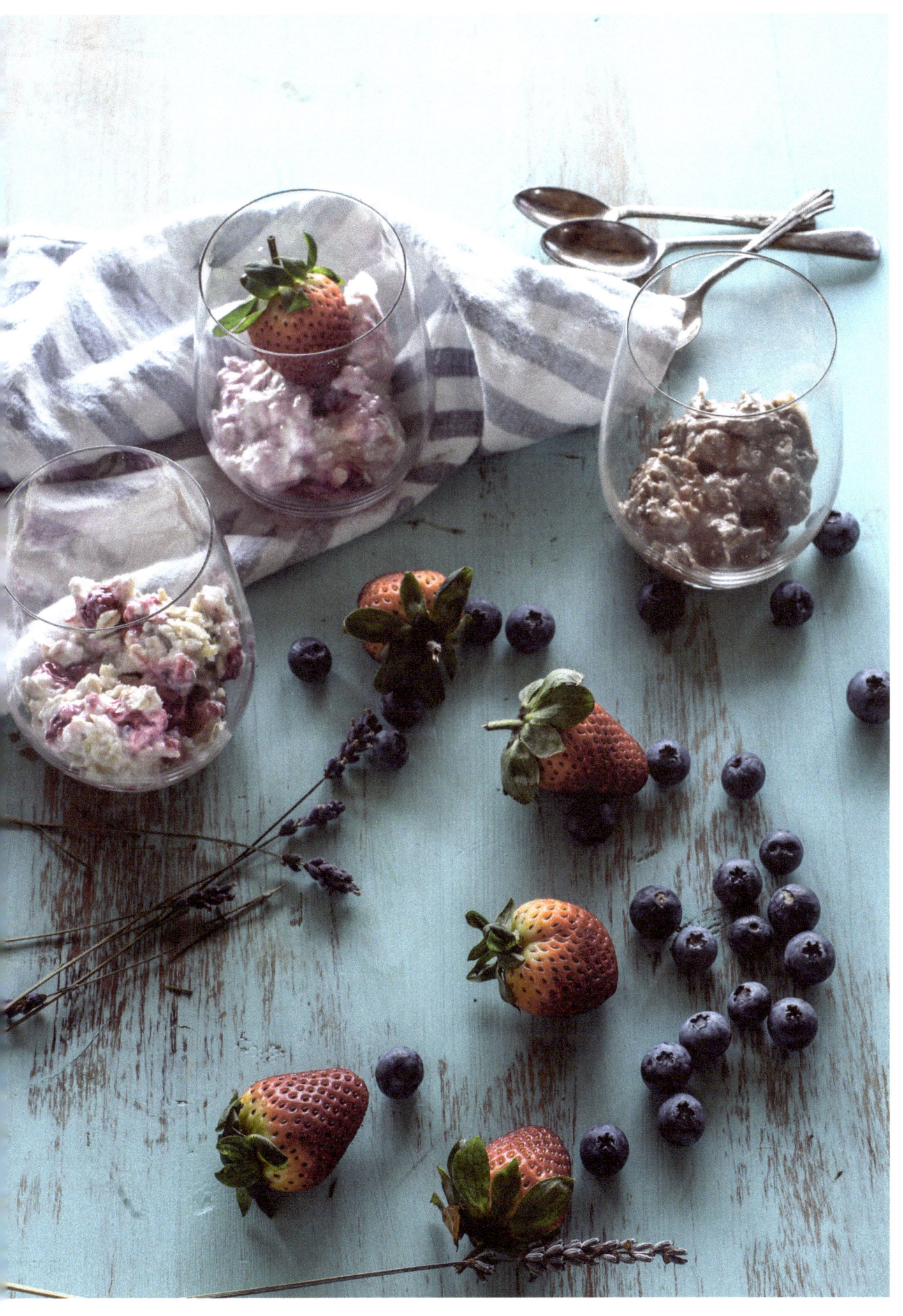

Baked Beans

SERVES 12

A great use for the ham bone when you have finished with the ham. The ham bone adds a great flavour to the beans. If you don't have a slow cooker you can braise these beans in the oven in a covered casserole dish for about four hours at 170°C. Please note that there can be a huge difference in cooking times in slow-cookers, I was surprised when I broke one my new one takes twice as long to cook on high as the old one, and taking the lid off to often will lengthen the cooking time. So, get to know your own.

1 dry cup beans, cannellini, blackeye, red kidney or a mixture

2 large carrots

2 sticks celery

2 bay leaf

1 cup chicken or vegetable stock

1 large onion

2 large cloves garlic

2 rashers bacon (or a ham hock or ham bone)

800 grams crushed tomato

1 teaspoon sweet paprika

½ teaspoon cumin

½ teaspoon ground coriander

2 tablespoons maple syrup

salt and pepper

robust extra virgin olive oil to serve

Cover the beans with water and leave to soak overnight.

Drain and put in the slow cooker with the peeled and finely diced carrot, bay leaves, stock, peeled and diced onion, crushed garlic, finely sliced bacon, tomato, paprika, cumin, coriander, maple syrup and salt and pepper and the ham if you are using it.

Cook for 4-7 hours on high or until the beans are well cooked and they are in a nice thick tomato sauce. If you are using ham it should pull apart off the bone.

Season with salt and pepper add serve.

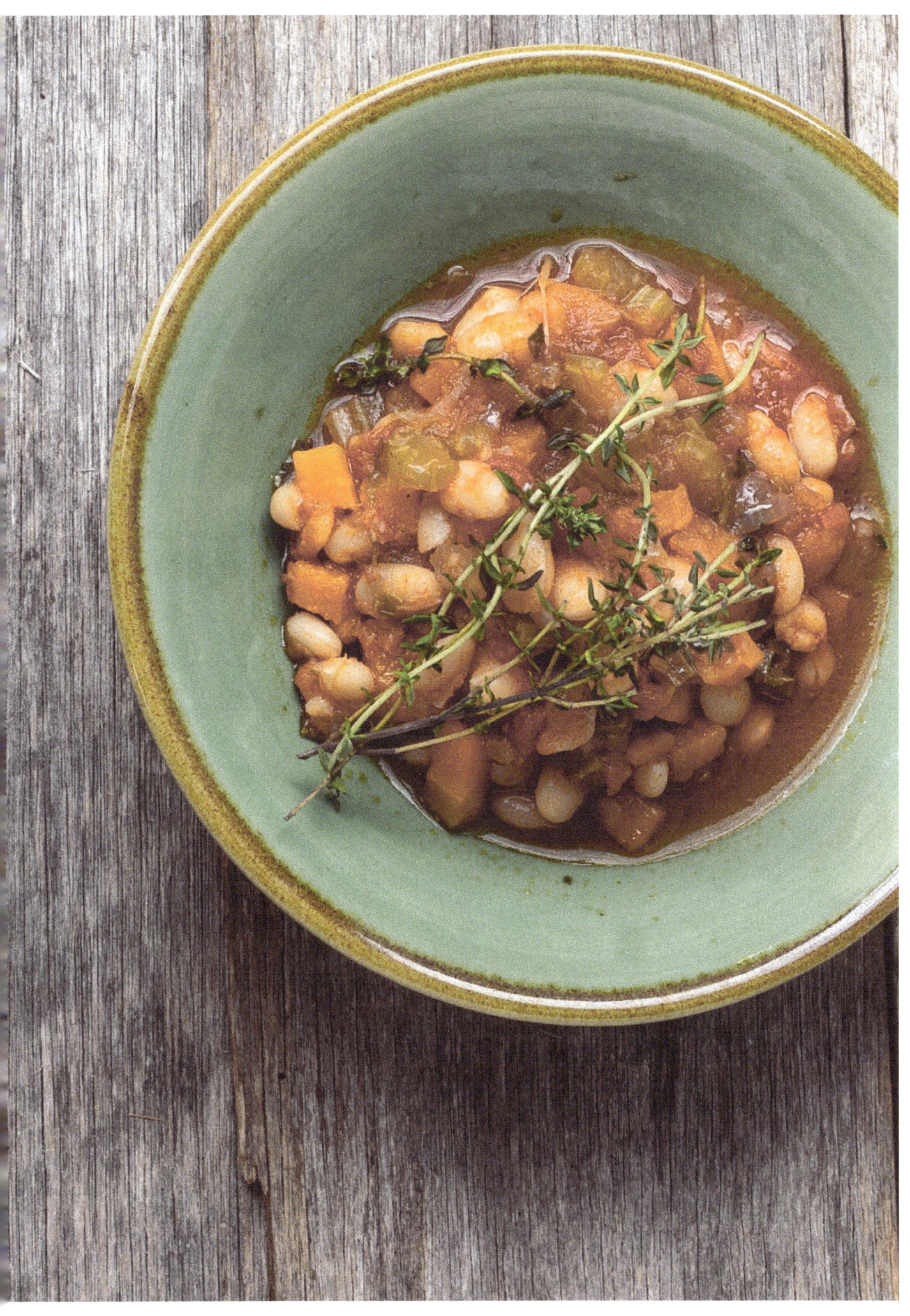

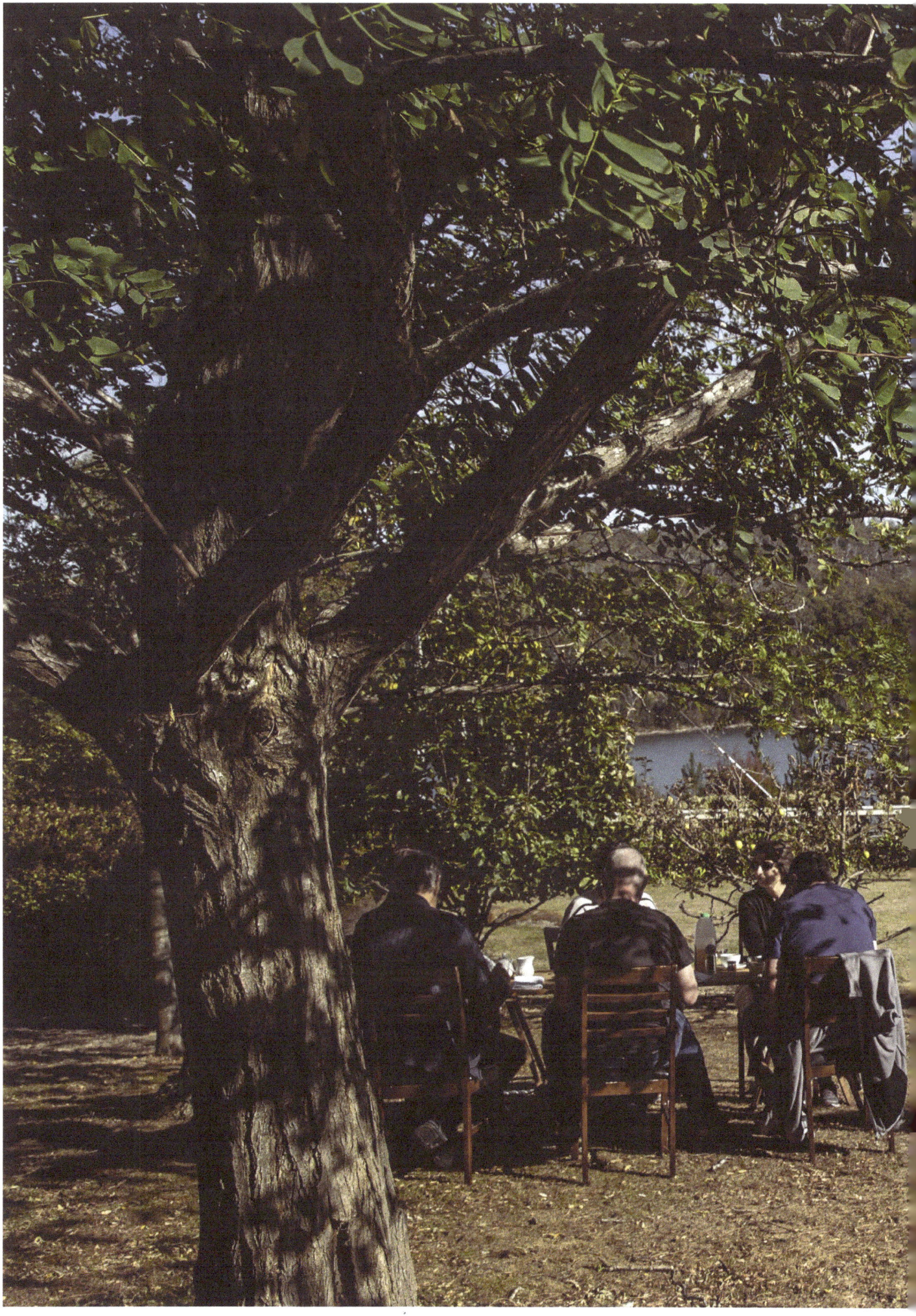

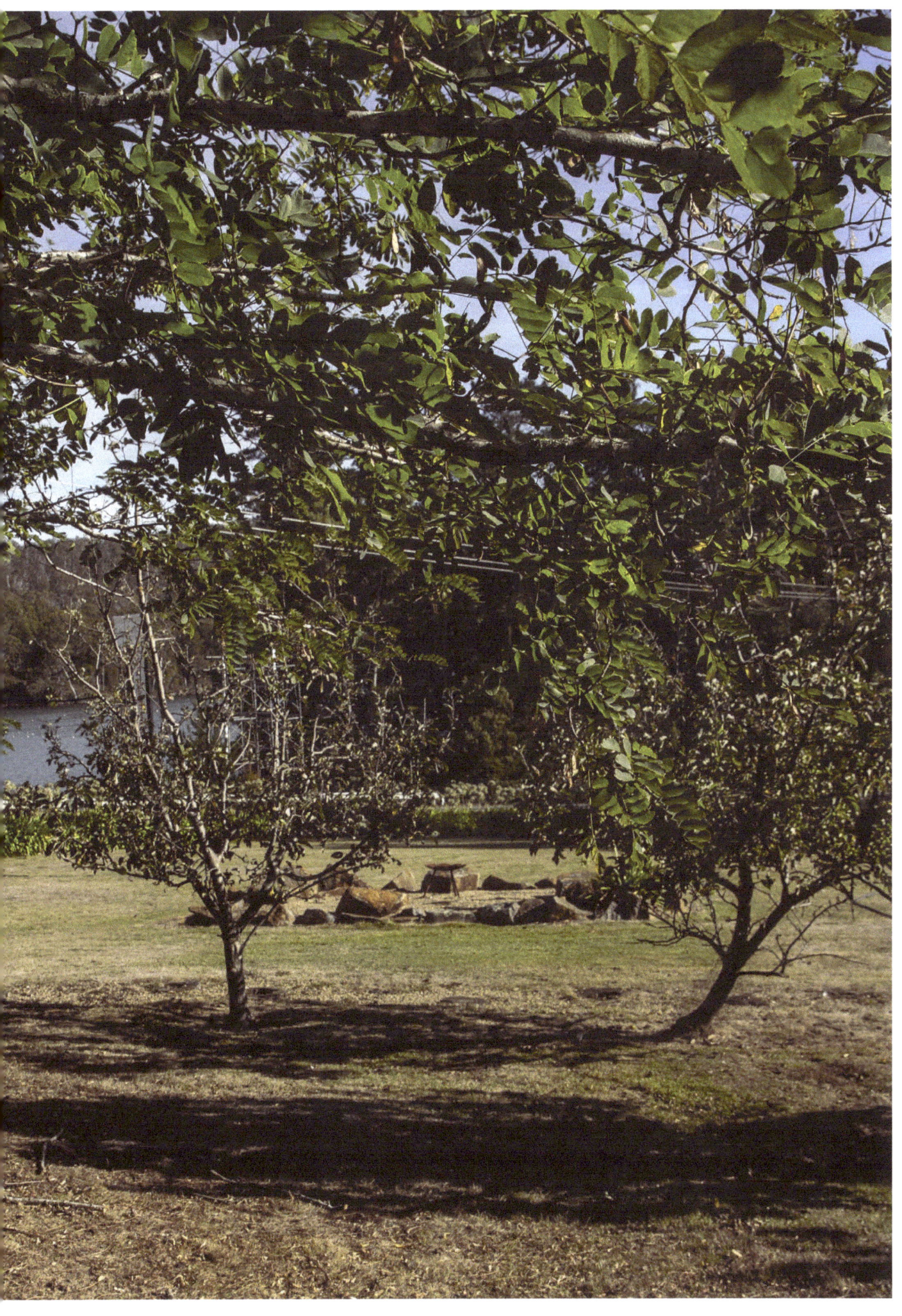

Chicken and Corn Soup

SERVES AT LEAST 10

This is another staple weeknight dinner or thermos in lunch box meal packed with veggies, many variations can be made. I have included it in this book as its one of the most popular recipe ideas I have shared on my website and social media for busy parents, easy, veggie packed and delicious! I don't know what facts have been proven by eating chicken soup when you are sick but are grandmothers were certainly onto something as the smell of a stock bubbling away inside on a cold winters day is mood uplifting to start with.

STOCK

1 Nichols free range chicken

Use the trimmings of the vegetables listed below that you have collected while cooking and have frozen, as I suggest in my stock making.

2 onions

3 sticks celery

3 carrot

1 leek

3 sprigs parsley

3 sprigs thyme

3 bay leaf

peppercorn

SOUP

3 carrots

3 onions

3 sticks celery

6 cloves garlic

½ large red chilli

1 teaspoon ginger

1 tablespoon robust extra virgin olive oil

2 cobs corn

2 tablespoons soy sauce

noodles or rice

green fresh veggies or frozen peas

To make the stock I use the slow cooker. Place the chicken in the slow cooker with the onion, celery, carrot, leek, parsley, thyme, bay leaf and peppercorn. Leave to cook for around 4 hours - the chicken should be thoroughly cooked and the stock fragrant.

Strain the stock off and set aside, discarding the veggie scraps, and remove the meat from the bones of the chicken.

To make the soup, finely dice the carrot, onion, celery, dice the garlic, chilli, ginger and remove the kernels from the cobs and blend the corn.

In a large heavy based pot heat the oil and sauté the carrot, onion, celery, garlic, chilli and ginger for a few minutes until softened. Add the stock and cook for around 20 minutes. Add the meat, green vegetables and noodles and season with the soy and pepper.

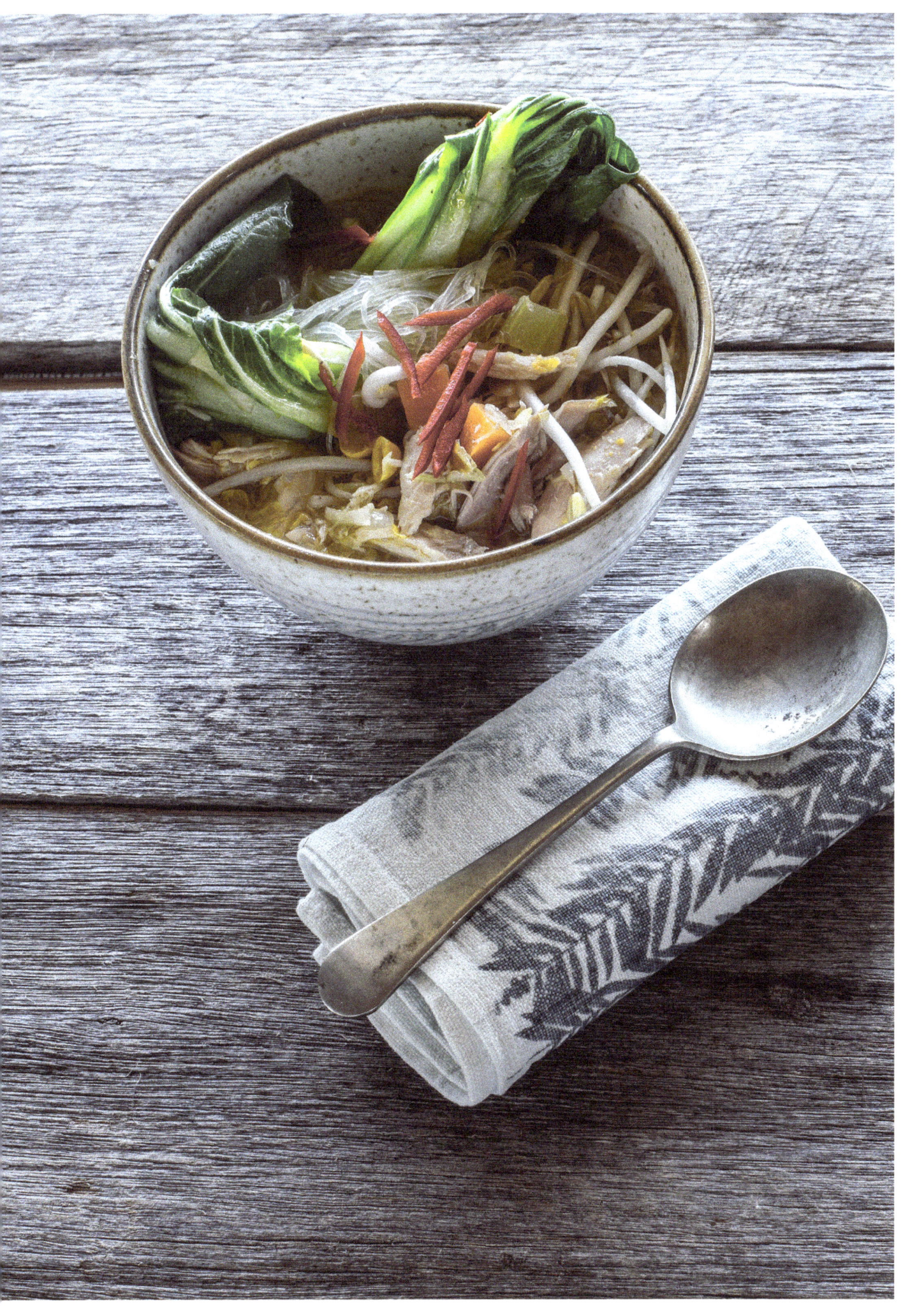

Chicken Minestrone

SERVES AT LEAST 10

A variation of this soup is eaten pretty much every week at our house. Packed with veggies it freezes well. Keep your cuttings from your cooking in a freezer bag in the freezer so it's easy to pop a stock into the slow cooker or pot. Save the whole veggies for the dishes you will consume! This makes a base soup I will split into 2-3 to freeze, reheat on busy weeknights maybe add some pasta or fresh, frozen or canned veggies. When re-heating the soup after freezing, season well with a good pinch of sea salt and pepper and a dump of robust herbaceous peppery extra virgin olive oil to liven up the flavours.

STOCK

1 chicken

1 leek

1 brown onion

2 carrots

2 sticks celery

3 sprigs parsley

3 sprigs thyme

3 bay leaves

10 peppercorns

SOUP

2 tablespoons extra virgin olive oil

2 onions

3 carrots

6 cloves garlic

4 sticks celery

800 grams tomato

3 tablespoon basil

3 tablespoon oregano

TO SERVE

1-2 cups of veggies per person such as beans, corn, peas, cabbage, broccoli, spinach, cauliflower, tins of beans frozen peas and corn.

To make the stock put the chicken in the slow cooker with the veggies and herbs or the trimmings from your freezer that you are replacing them with.

Cook for 4 hours or until the chicken is cooked. Strain the stock into a container and remove all the meat from the chicken.

To make the soup, peel the carrots and dice into a 5mm cube, peel and finely dice the onion, dice the celery, purée the tomato, peel and crush the garlic.

In a large heavy based pot, heat the extra virgin olive oil, add the onion, carrot, celery and garlic and sauté until soft. Add the stock, herbs and tomato and simmer for 20 minutes.

Add the shredded chicken meat and 1-2 cups of veggies per person, that you have on hand (veggies from the fridge freezer and pantry or cooked pasta).

Serve with crusty bread and robust extra virgin olive oil.

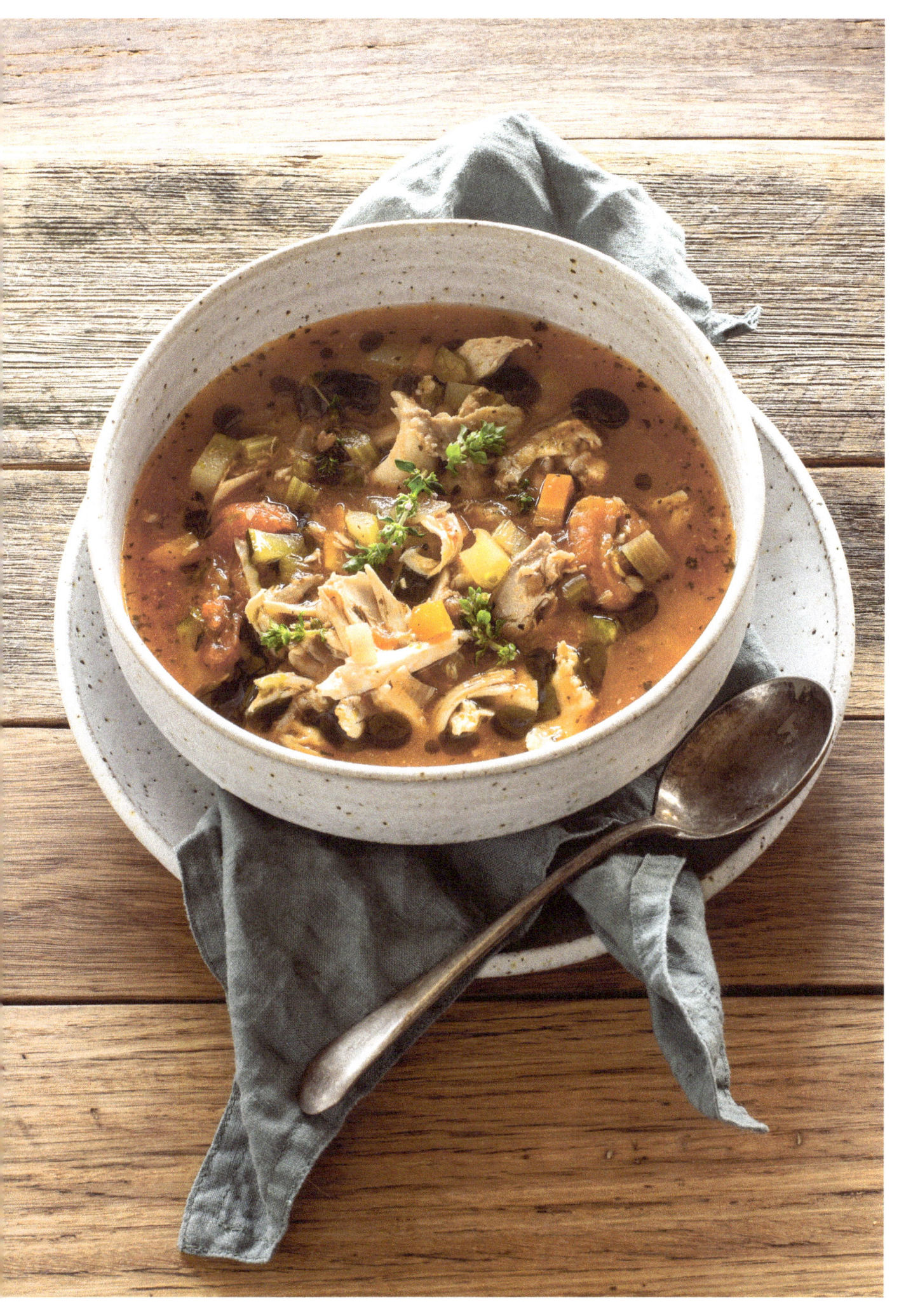

Smoked Oyster Pate

MAKES A DECENT SIZE POT

2 dozen angasi or pacific oysters

dash extra virgin olive oil

½ small onion

1 clove garlic

½ teaspoon fennel seed

100ml cream

pinch pepper

BRINE MIX

1 tablespoon brown sugar

1 tablespoon salt

1 cup water

Split the oysters and remove the meat. The oysters need to cure overnight in the brine mix which is the brown sugar, salt and water. Also soak your smoking wood chips overnight so they don't burn.

If you don't have a smoker, you can use a steamer pot or a pot with a raised rack inside, and a lid. You just need to be able to place the oysters above the wood chips and keep the smoke surrounding them.

Line the bottom of the pot with foil and place the wood chips that have been soaked overnight on top of the foil. Place the pot on a burner (side of the barbeque?) outside until the wood chips are smokey. Place the oysters on the steaming pot or rack and put the lid on. The oysters will take about 10 minutes to be smoked and cooked through.

To make the pate, in a small heavy based pot or your thermocooker, sauté the garlic and onion with the ground fennel seed until soft and fragrant. Add the cream and oysters and then bring back to the boil. Purée and then season with salt and pepper.

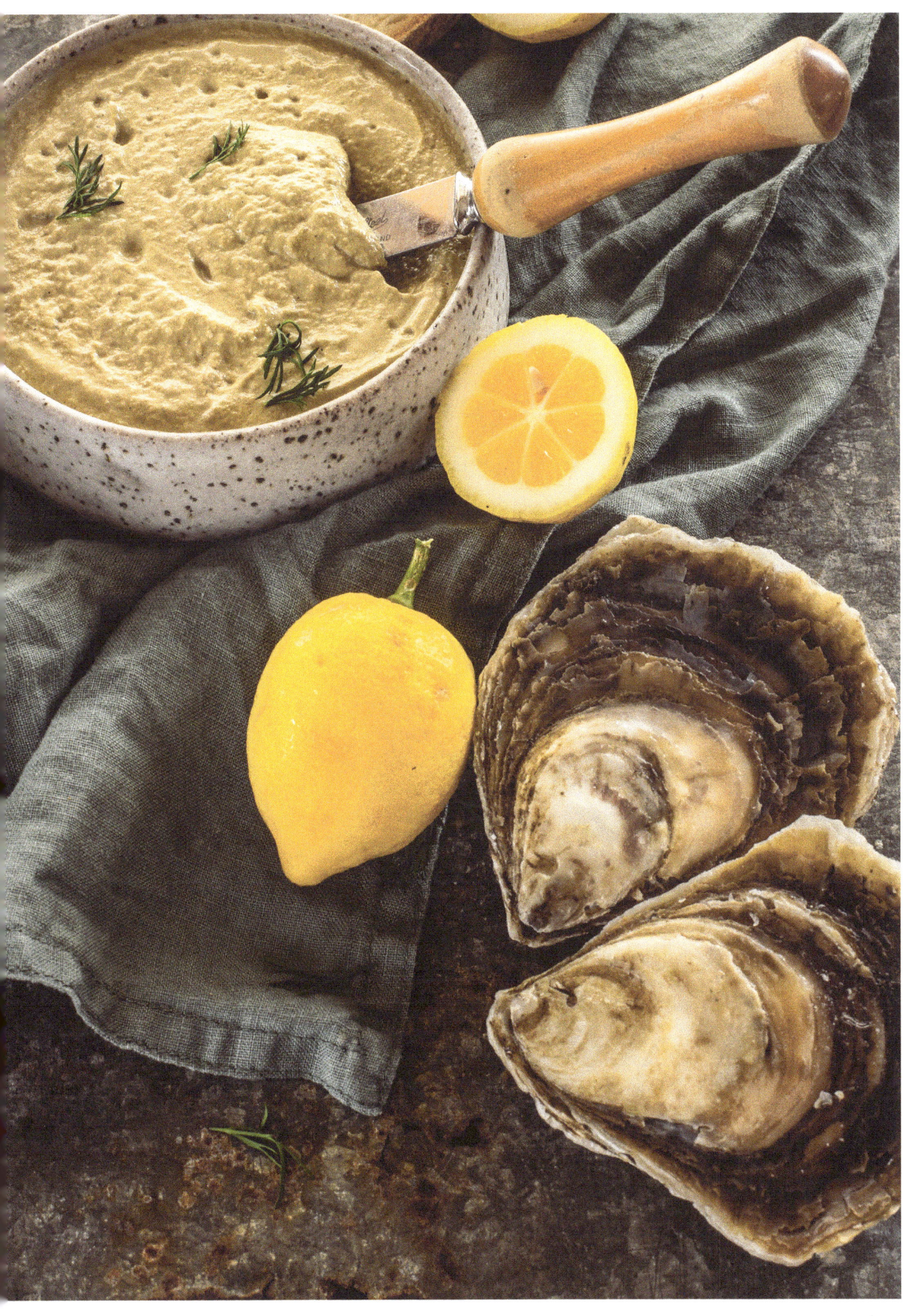

Abalone Confit

SERVES 4 AS AN ENTREE

Abalone, for us, is normally cooked when freshly caught and then shared over a few drinks whilst camping with friends or family - its never really served on a dish in a restaurant! This is one of my favourite ways to cook abalone. You can turn this into a fancy entree or meal by serving with a tasty salad or some crusty bread or grissini to dip into the gorgeous oil you cooked the abalone in.

abalone

extra virgin olive oil

sea salt

Shuck the abalone from the shell by cutting as close to the shell as you can and remove the guts. It's up to you if you want to eat the black lip or not, I personally don't waste it as it might be a little tougher, but still tasty.

Wrap the abalone in a clean cloth. This will help you for grip and also so you don't make a massive mess. Bash a few times with a meat mallet to tenderise it. In a small heavy based pan, put the abalone large foot side down and just cover with a delicate in flavour extra virgin olive oil. Cook for approximately one hour, keeping the temperature below 90°C.

Serve the abalone cold, warm or hot with plenty of sea salt.

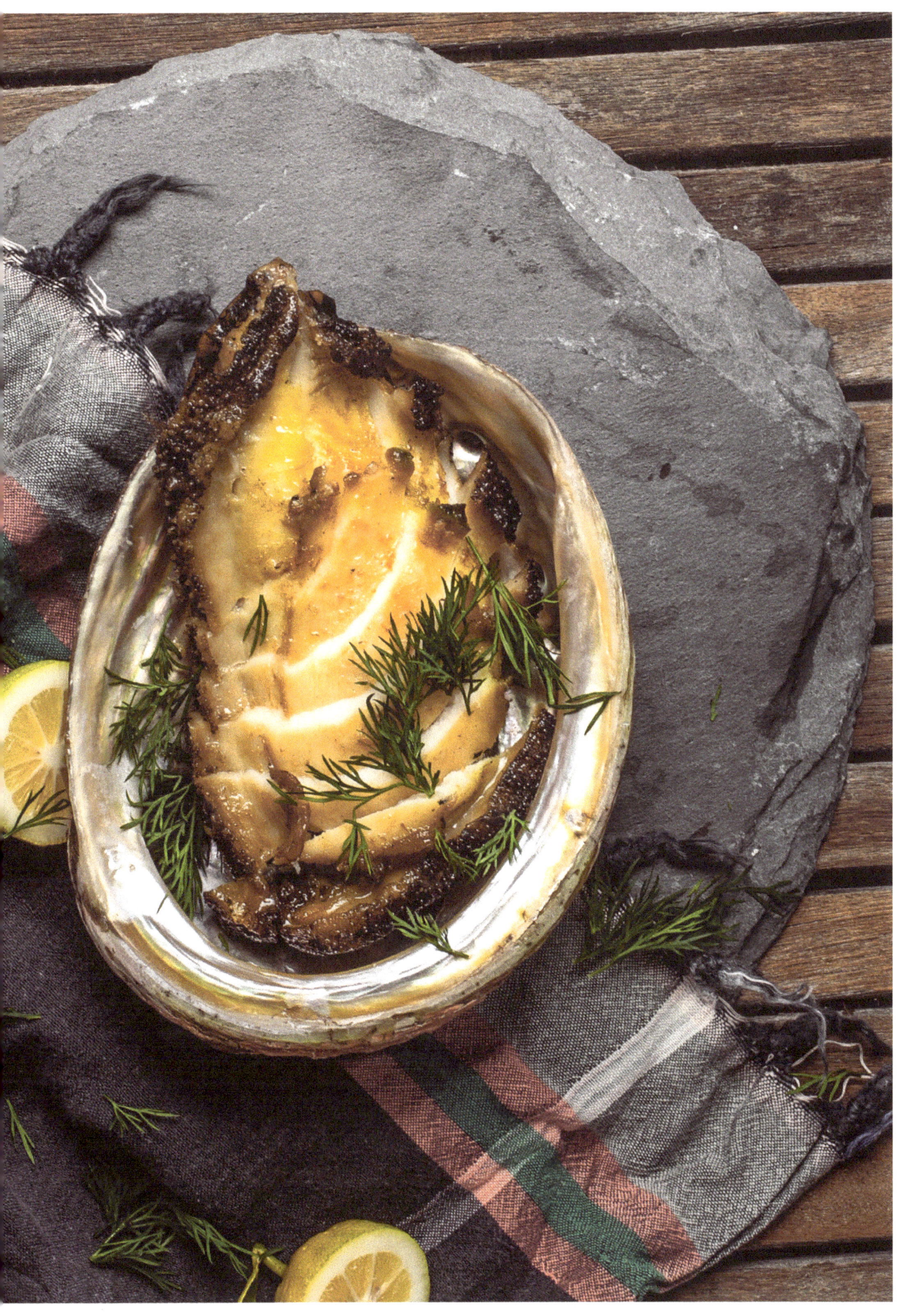

Chicken Liver Pate

MAKES 4 SMALL POTS

1 tablespoon butter

500 grams chicken livers

1 rasher bacon

1 small onion

1 clove garlic

1 teaspoon dried basil

½ teaspoon dried thyme

100ml cream

shot brandy

white pepper

sea salt

extra virgin olive oil to top and store

In a heavy based pan or your thermocooker, sauté the butter, chopped bacon, peeled and chopped onion, peeled and chopped garlic and sauté until soft and fragment

Add the livers and herbs and sauté over a low heat until just cooked. Add the brandy and cream and bring to the boil.

Purée and place in pots, top with a thin layer of extra virgin olive oil to set in the refrigerator.

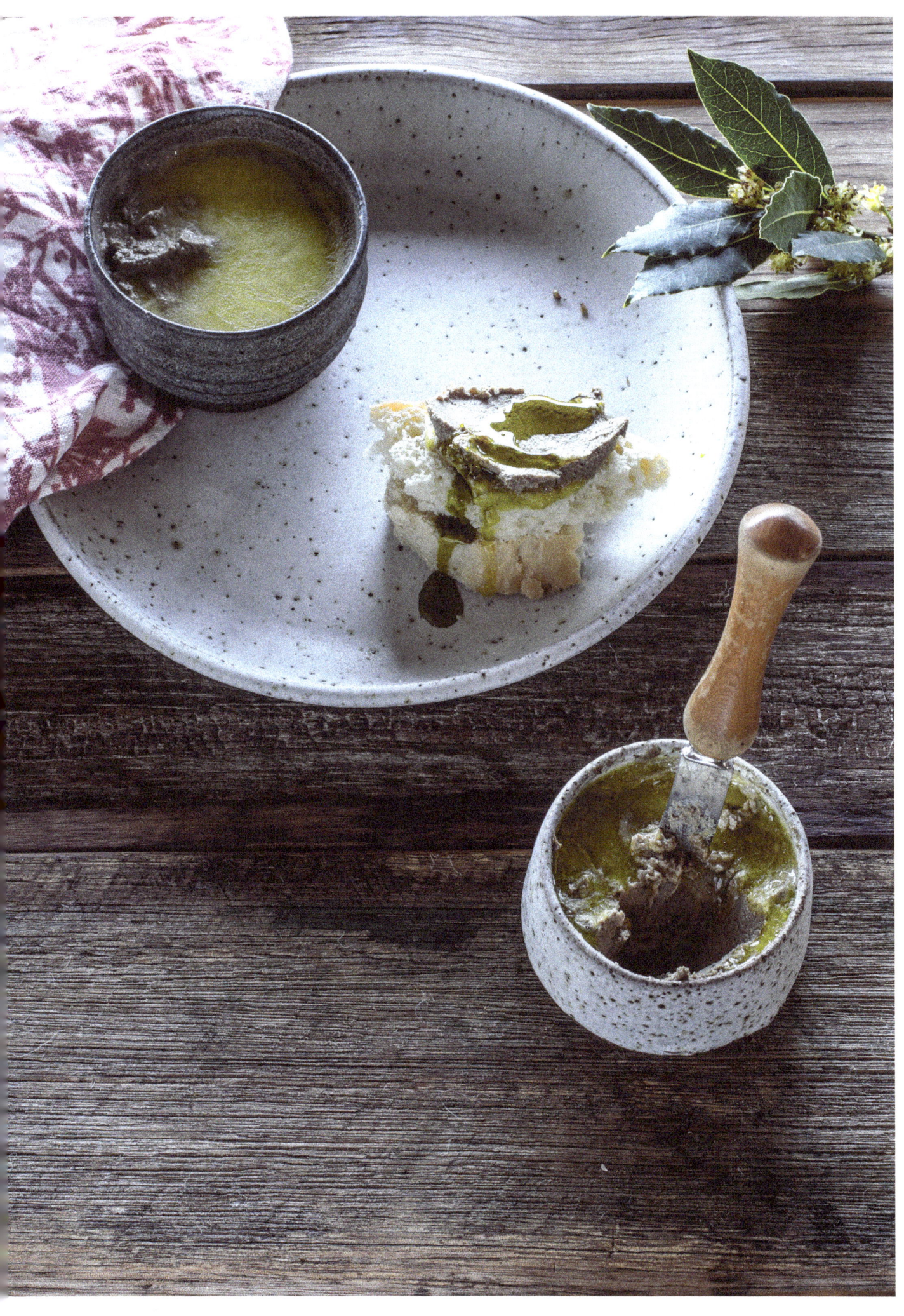

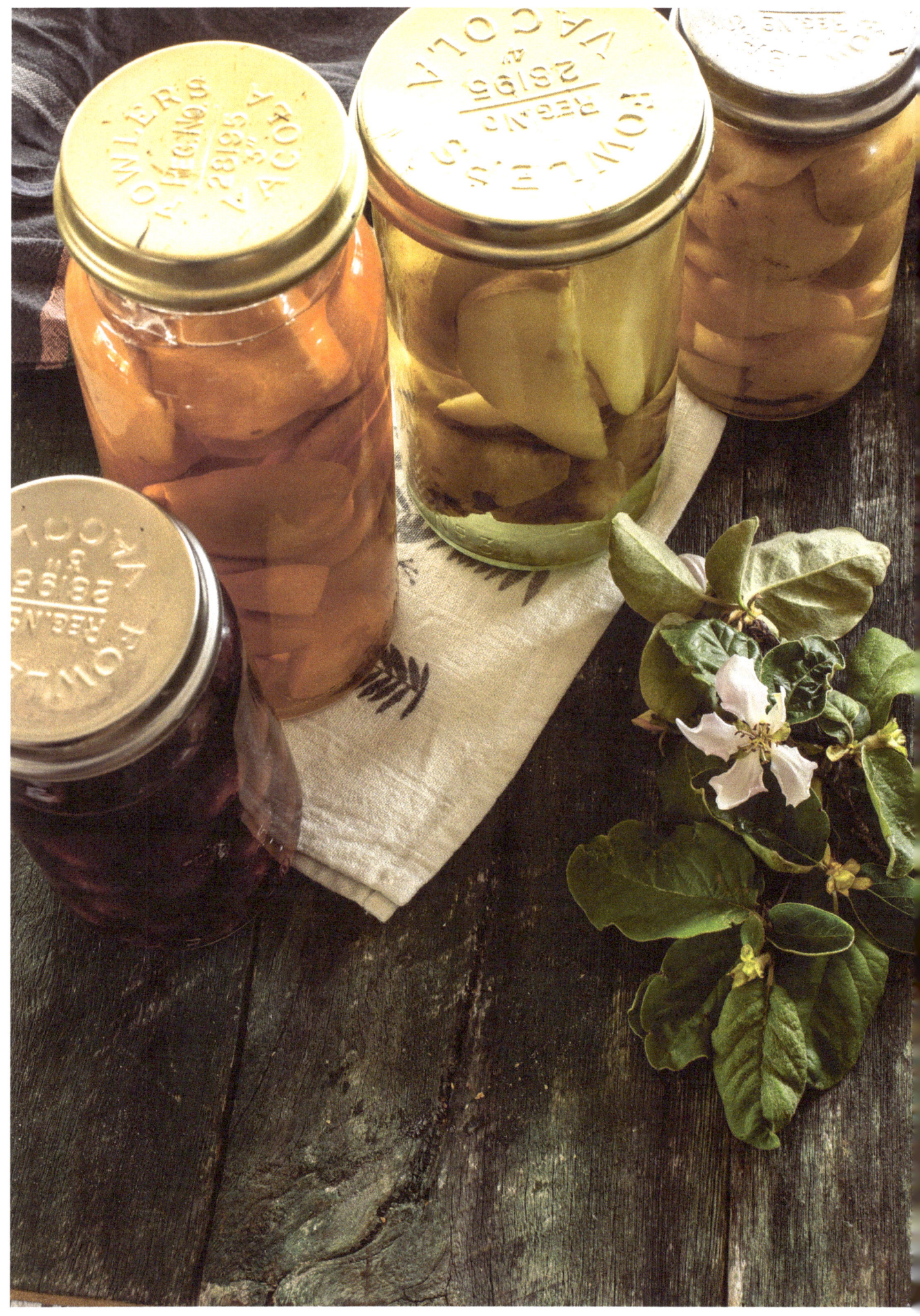

"Preserving food is easy to do, and the benefits of having home-produced foods in the pantry far outweighs the effort you put in."

Beef Marinated in Wild Pepper Isle's Tasmanian Pepper Berry Soy served with a Thai Noodle Salad

SERVES AT LEAST 2

1 Summerlea Farm beef ribeye

MARINADE

2 tablespoons Wild Pepper Isle Tasmanian Pepper Berry Soy

1 tablespoon robust extra virgin olive oil

SALAD

2 bok choy

1 carrot

⅛ cup bean sprouts

1 red capsicum

2 cups cooked rice noodles

bunch coriander

bunch mint

1 oak lettuce

DRESSING

1 tablespoon Wild Pepper Isle Tasmanian Pepper Berry Soy

2 cloves garlic

2 tablespoons lime juice

Marinate the steak for a few hours before cooking in the soy and oil that has been mixed well together.

Clean and chop the bok choy, peel and cut the carrot into skinny batons, slice capsicum and pick the herbs, wash and spin the lettuce leaves, add the spouts and cooled cooked rice noodles and toss gently and assemble on a platter.

To cook the steak, heat a barbeque or pan, add the steak and brown on both sides well then turn the temperature down to a medium high heat until it is cooked to your liking (rest wrapped in foil for at least 10 minutes before serving).

Mix the dressing ingredients together well and dress the salad, serve immediately.

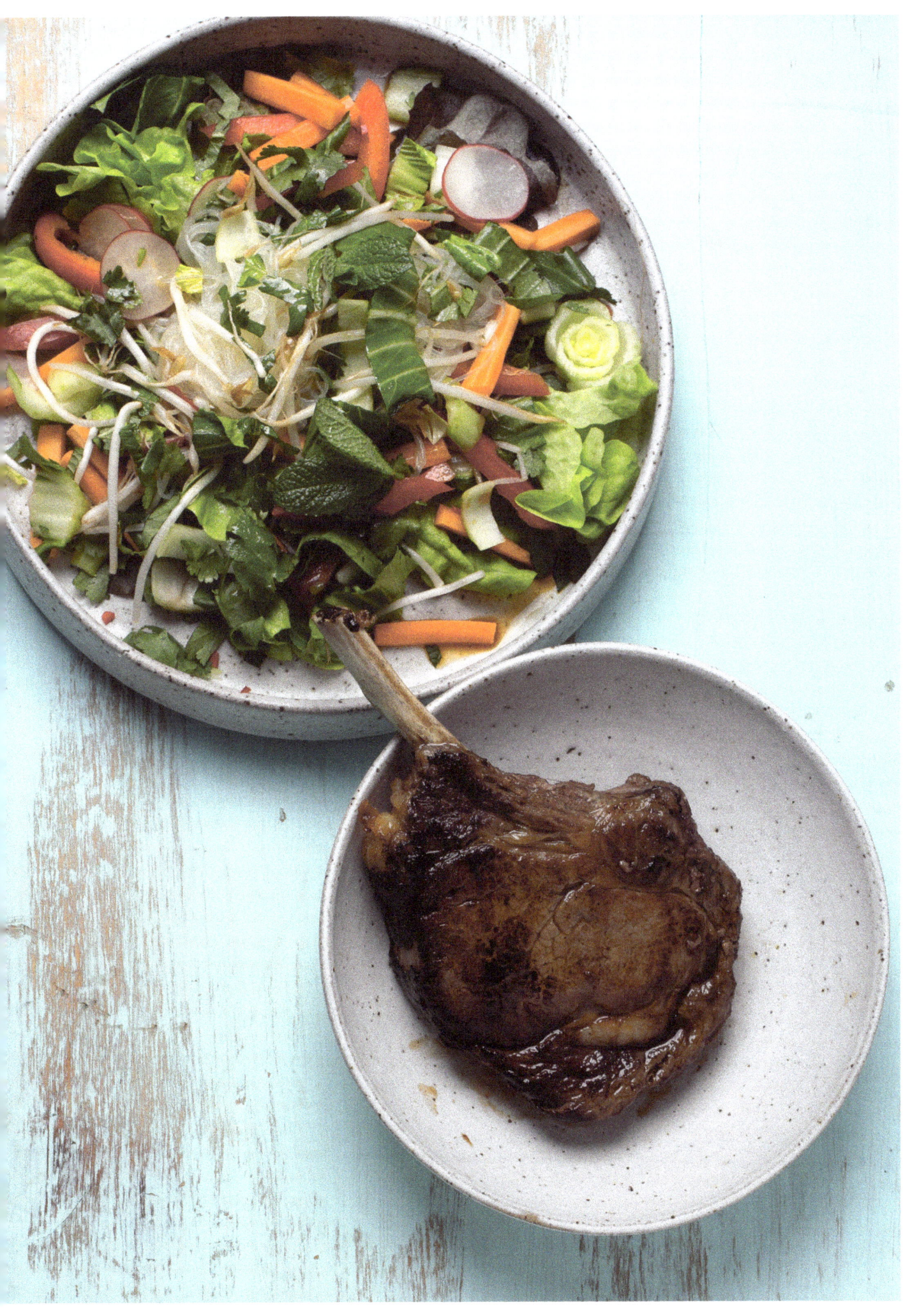

Rhubarb Cream Brulée

SERVES 4

Cream brulée is one of the simplest impressive dessert. Basically, a baked custard with a crispy toffee top. The brulée can be made with loads of different fruits and flavour combinations using rhubarb, apples, berries, lavender and more. Make the brulée early on the day of serving to simply crisp up the sugar on top to serve.

200ml milk

200ml cream

50 grams sugar

5 egg yolks

3 sticks rhubarb

Heat the oven to 150°C.

To lightly stew the rhubarb simply chop it into battons and place into a pot on the stove with a dash of water and cook over a low heat for around 6 minutes until soft. To make the brulée, bring the milk and cream to a gentle simmer on the stove and then turn off.

While the milk and cream is on the stove mix the yolks and sugar together well with a whisk in a large bowl, pour in the warm milk mix while whisking continuously. In the bottom of four ramekins place the stewed rhubarb and then pour the mix over.

Place the ramekins in a water bath into a baking tray with the water coming at least halfway up the side of the ramekin.

Place the tray in the oven for around 20 minutes until they are just set.

They can now be served warm or cooled to serve.

To create the crisp toffee top simply sprinkle over caster sugar and cook gently using a circular motion for an even cook with the kitchen blow torch.

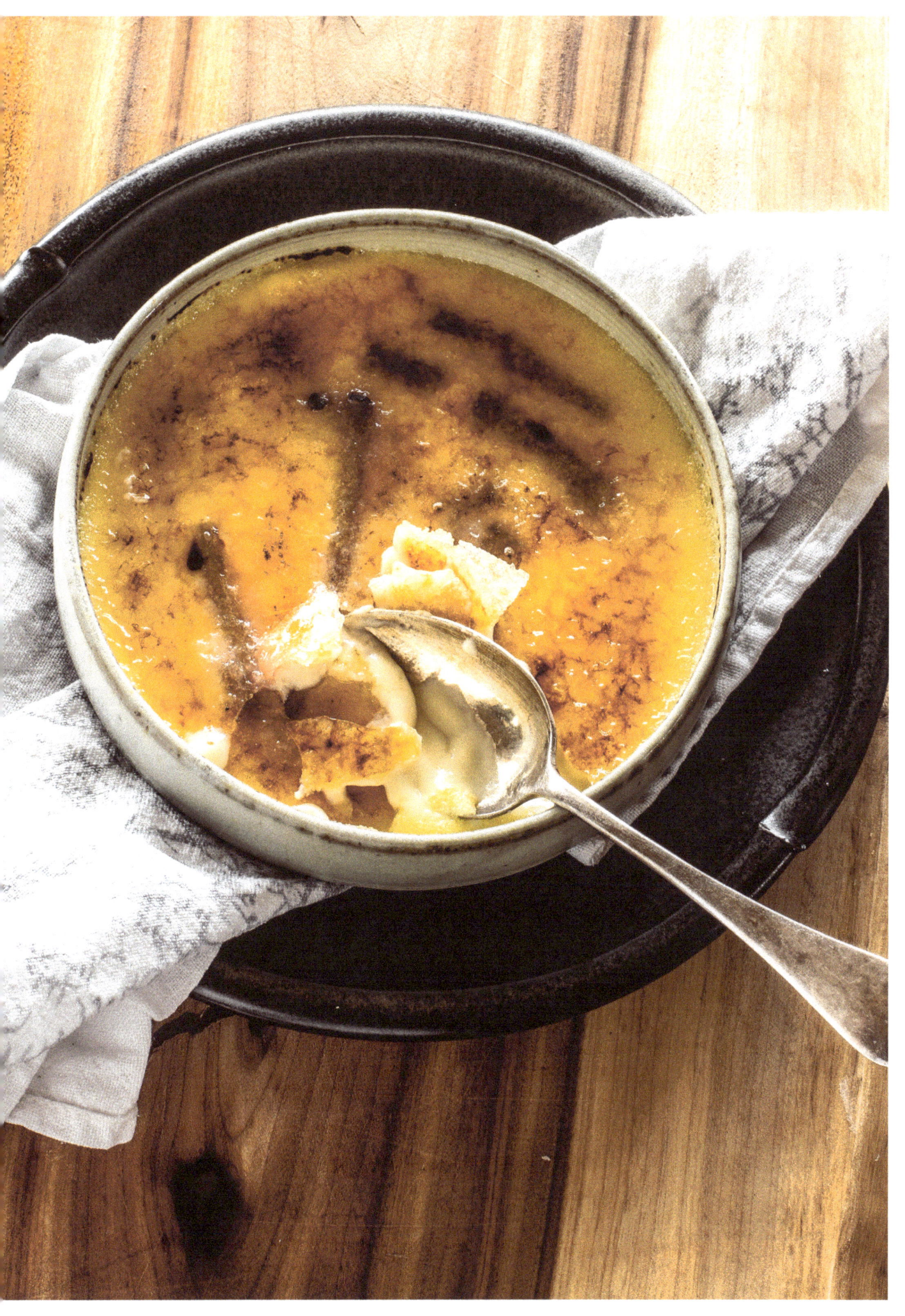

Pickled Octopus

MAKES 2 OR 3 JARS

I love some pickled octopus in the refrigerator for a delicious and quick lunch protein with a simple salad, it also makes a pretty fancy canape.

1 kilo octopus tentacles
250ml white wine vinegar
250ml red wine vinegar
20 peppercorns
6 bay leaves
2 tablespoons fennel seed
6 cloves garlic
8 sprigs oregano
extra virgin olive oil

Bring a large pot of salted water to the boil and cook the tentacles for around 10 minutes until cooked through. Remove the tentacles from the pot and slice across the tentacles in 4mm thickness to create thin discs of octopus.

Fill small sterilised preserving jars with the octopus. Place the vinegar in a pot and bring it to the boil. Distribute the herbs, garlic and pepper between the jars and pour in the vinegar top with the olive oil.

Seal the lids and boil in the preserving unit or water bath for 20 minutes. Store in the fridge for a few weeks.

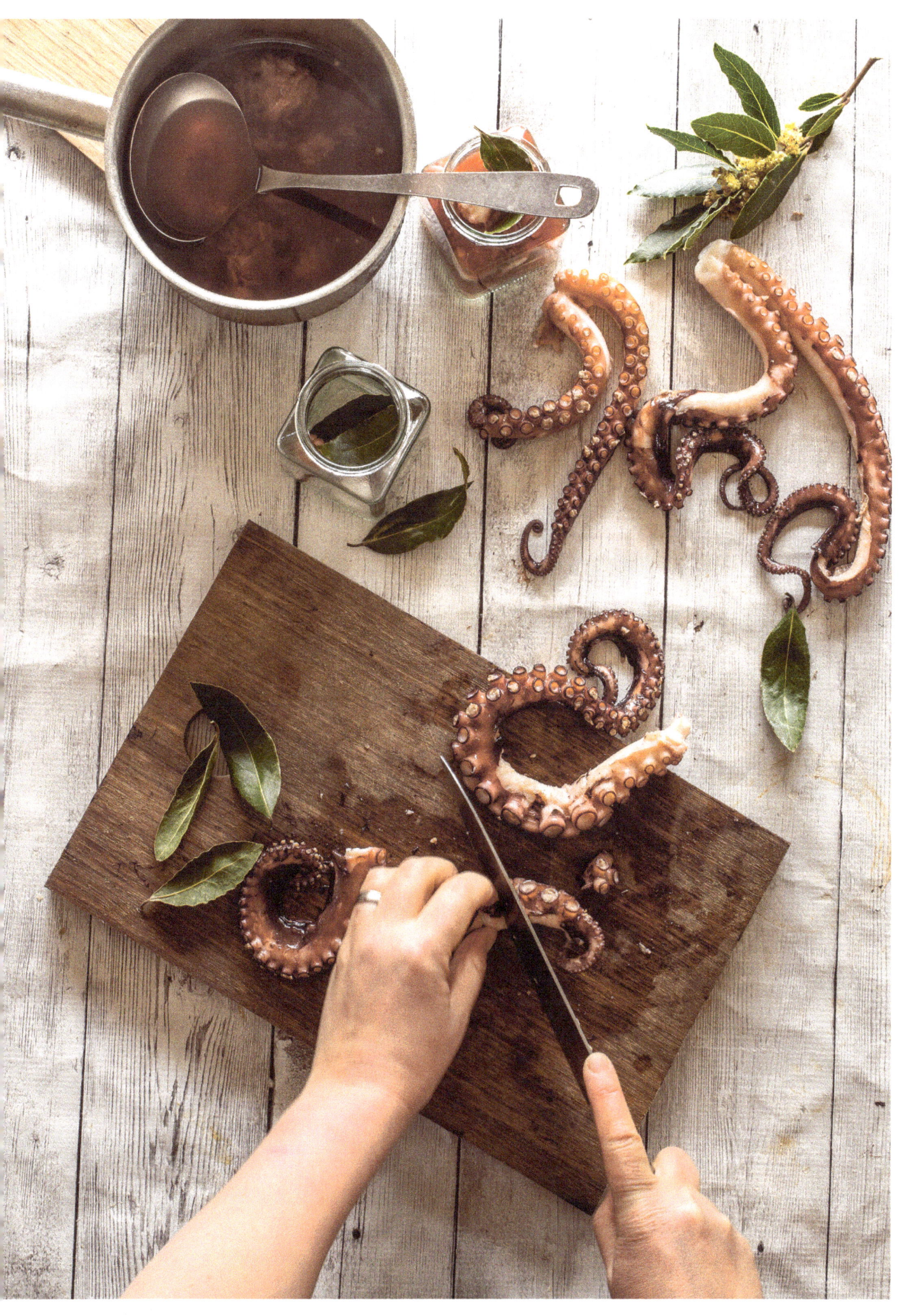

Lamb Kashmir Korma

SERVES 6

I was once employed as the head chef at a popular bar and for whatever reason the manager insisted there be a curry on the specials menu at all times. So I had a lot of fun creating lots of delicious curries while working there. Now as a busy mum of three young kids, I appreciate how super handy in the home kitchen a curry can be, as leaving a curry in the fridge for a few days only improves the flavour. Make on the weekend for a quick and easy weeknight meal.

500 grams lamb

2 cups natural yogurt

½ teaspoon Campo De Flori saffron threads

1 onion

¼ teaspoon turmeric

1 teaspoon dried chilli

½ teaspoon ginger

½ teaspoon cinnamon

½ teaspoon cumin

½ teaspoon coriander

½ teaspoon white pepper

½ teaspoon fennel

2 cups beef stock

TO SERVE

rice and greens or naan bread

Roast your dried spices over a low heat on a pan until fragrant and aromatic. Cool and blend with the onion, saffron and yogurt (I use my thermocooker). Mix in the diced lamb and leave at least overnight.

I use the slow cooker but you could use a low 160°C oven with the curry in a baking dish with a lid, to braise this lamb for 2-3 hours. Place the lamb and stock in the slow cooker and cook on high for 4-5 hours until the meat is tender.

If you would like the sauce thicker, make a paste of equal parts plain flour and extra virgin olive oil and whisk this into the simmering sauce.

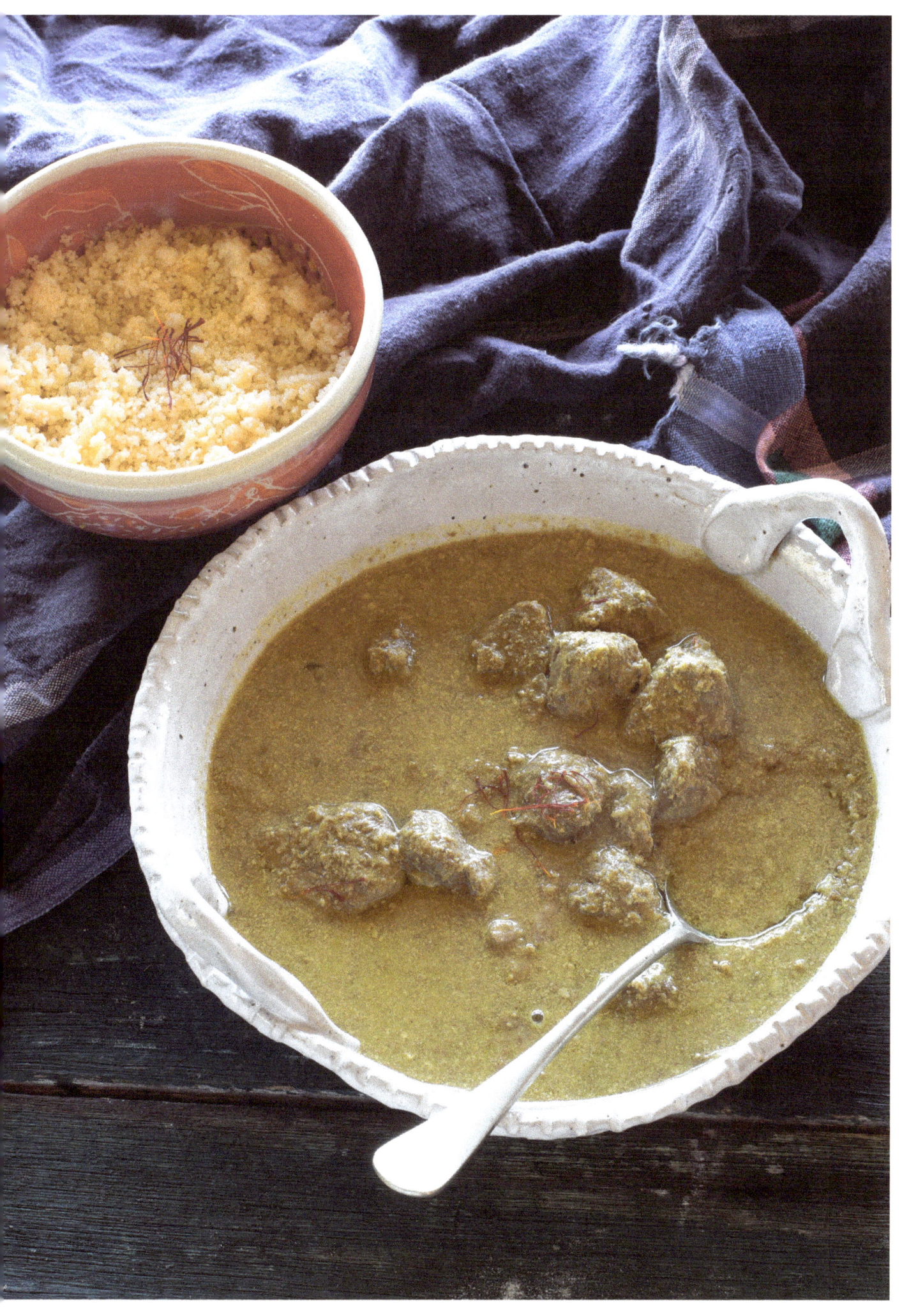

Salmon Carpaccio

SERVES 8 FOR AN ENTREE

This is a classic dish, best with the freshest seafood you can get your hands on! The ideas for flavouring are limitless - swap around different vinegar and oils and fresh herbs and condiments to serve with it - I change it up all the time - soy and lime works well too. How long you cure the seafood for is totally up to your personal preference. I have seen others marinate the seafood in the jars for days to fully cure. For delicious fresh Tassal salmon my choice would be no longer than five minutes as I don't want the salmon to cook at all and I still want to be able to taste the salmon. I cooked a version of this recipe at the Wooden Boat Festival Kitchen theatre with scallop meat roe on, and it was loved by the audience. The recipe is actually adapted from my book Seafood Every Day. In the book I serve it with oysters, you could let them cure for longer and cook the oysters. It really is the easiest no fuss but delicious and impressive entree or canapés for a dinner party!

400 grams salmon fillet, head or middle, where the fillet is fatter

2 tablespoons capers

2 tablespoons pickled cucumbers use a jar to keep it simple

60ml red wine vinegar

juice of one lemon

4 sprigs thyme

2 tablespoons olive oil

sea salt

cracked pepper

Slice the salmon into thin slices and lay onto plates. Sprinkle finely chopped capers, pickled cucumbers and herbs over the fish. Squeeze the lemon juice over and then drizzle the vinegar and oil.

Season with cracked pepper and sea salt.

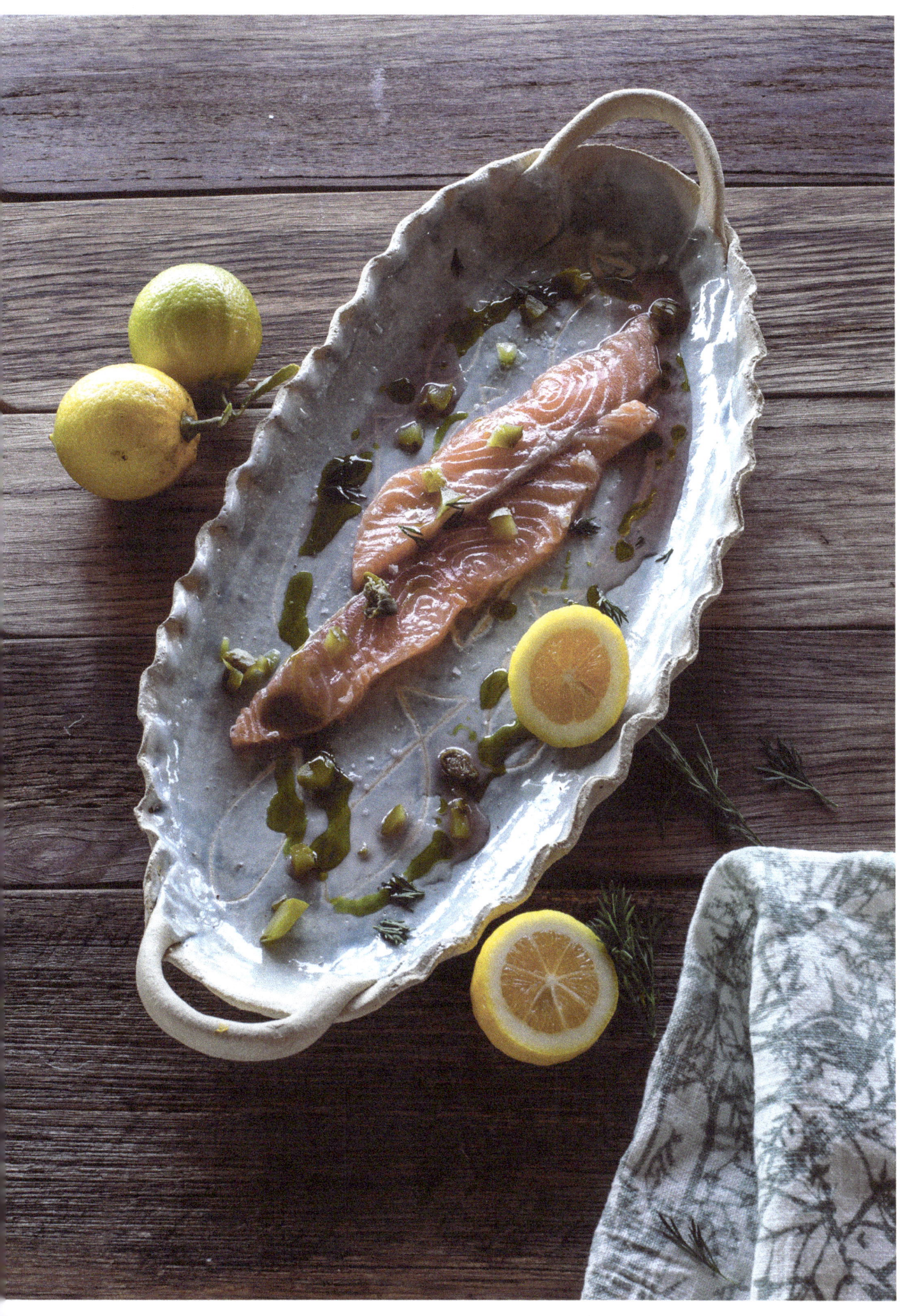

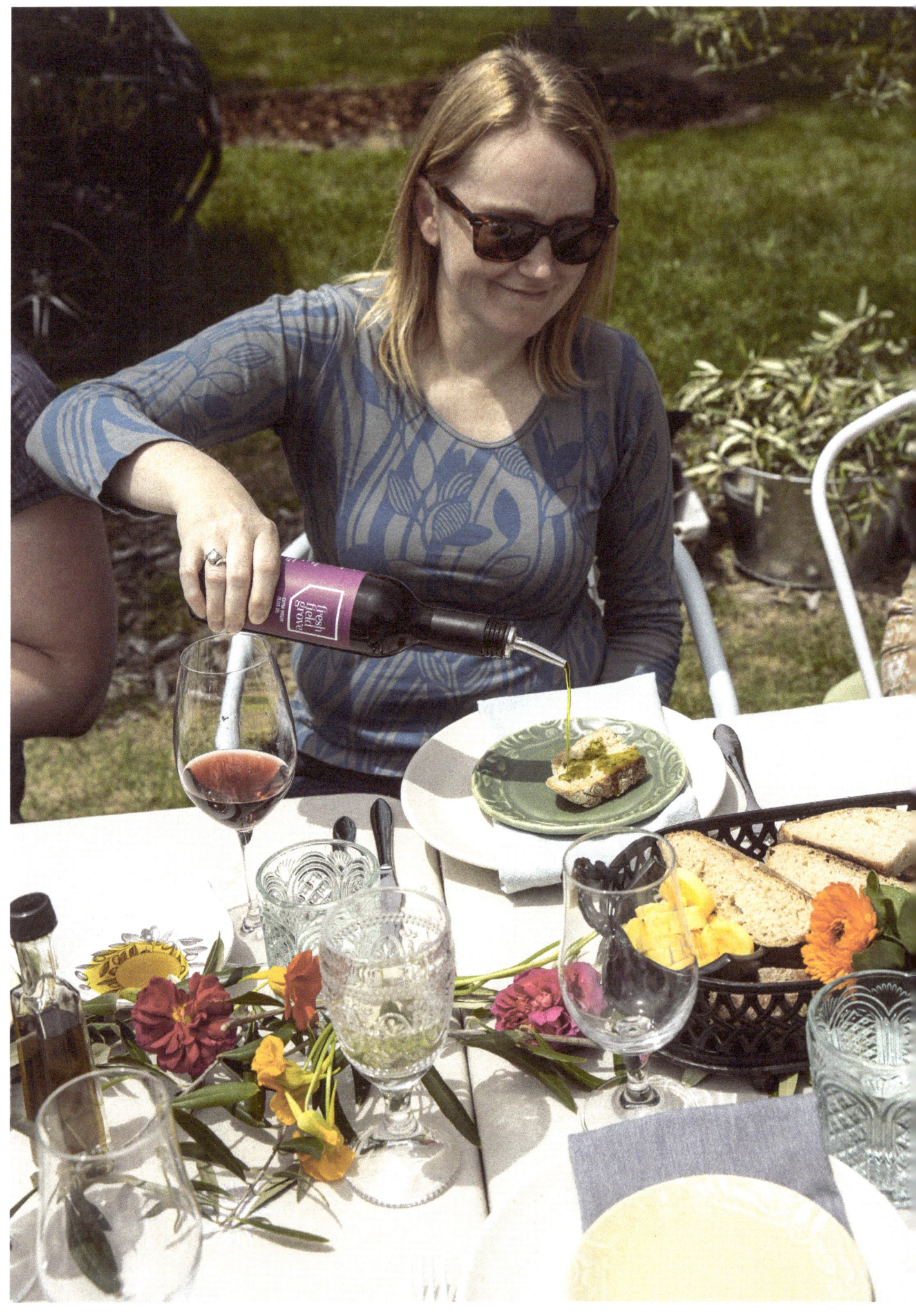

"The olive tree is surely the richest gift of Heaven"

THOMAS JEFFERSON

Taramasalata

MAKES 4 TUBS

I first learnt how to make taramasalata dip in an authentic Greek restaurant on the Hobart waterfront many years ago. Taramasalata is traditionally made from a salted cod roe paste called tarama. This tarama stuff generally comes in huge buckets imported from somewhere that would take you about 12 months in a commercial kitchen to use. If you've attended my workshops or been following me for a while on social media you'll know I am all about how to make things easy in the home kitchen and practical. What would you do with the other 400 tablespoon serves of tarama paste at the end of the recipe? And, of course, I always do like to support Tasmanian producers. This version uses salmon roe and hot smoked salmon - try to get the fatty middle bit of the hot smoked salmon side. Also, a great way to use up stale bread, I always pop the crusts in a bag in the freezer so I have some to make a dip like this or for bread crumbs or crusts.

100 grams salmon roe

150 grams Tassal hot smoked salmon

2 cloves garlic

juice of one lemon

1 tablespoon white wine vinegar

sea salt

pepper

4 slices bread into crumbs

approximately 300ml delicate or medium extra virgin olive oil

We are using the same emulsion style method to make this dip just like we would when making mayo or aioli. In the thermocooker or food processor add the salmon, roe, garlic, lemon juice, vinegar, salt, pepper and crumbs and blend until smooth.

Then add the oil in a slow drizzle while blending, stop and taste often until it becomes a smooth pink thick and creamy dip.

Season with salt and pepper. This is so good serve with home cut fat chips and battered fish or as a dip in the lunchboxes with fresh veggies sticks.

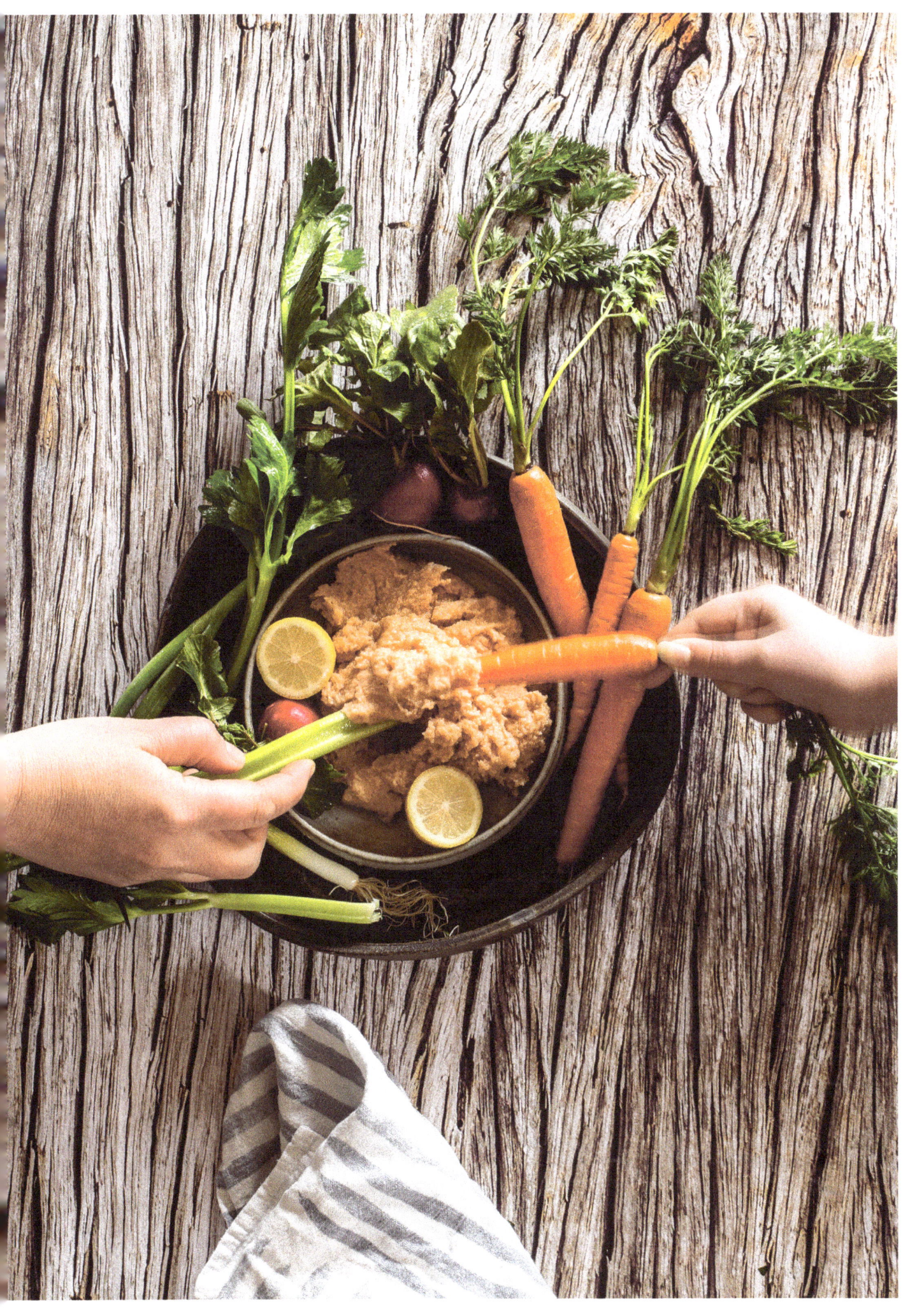

Jalapeño Bread

MAKES ONE LOAF

A great way to spice up a potentially boring meal such as a simple soup.

500 grams bakers flour

1 teaspoon bread improver

1 teaspoon salt

1 teaspoon sugar

1 teaspoon yeast

300ml - 320ml water

100 grams pickled jalapeño peppers

100 grams cheese

Heat the oven to 200°C.

To make the dough knead all ingredients well, I use the thermocooker to knead my dough for 2 minutes or you can use a mixer or knead by hand on the bench for around 10 minutes to produce a smooth firm dough. Cover and leave to rise in a warm position until the dough has doubled in size. Knock the dough back down and divide into 2 and roll into tight balls.

Roll each ball out and lay the peppers and the cheese over each and then roll each up into a loaf shape. Place on a baking tray and leave somewhere warm to double in size.

Bake for around 15-20 minutes or until golden brown and cooked through.

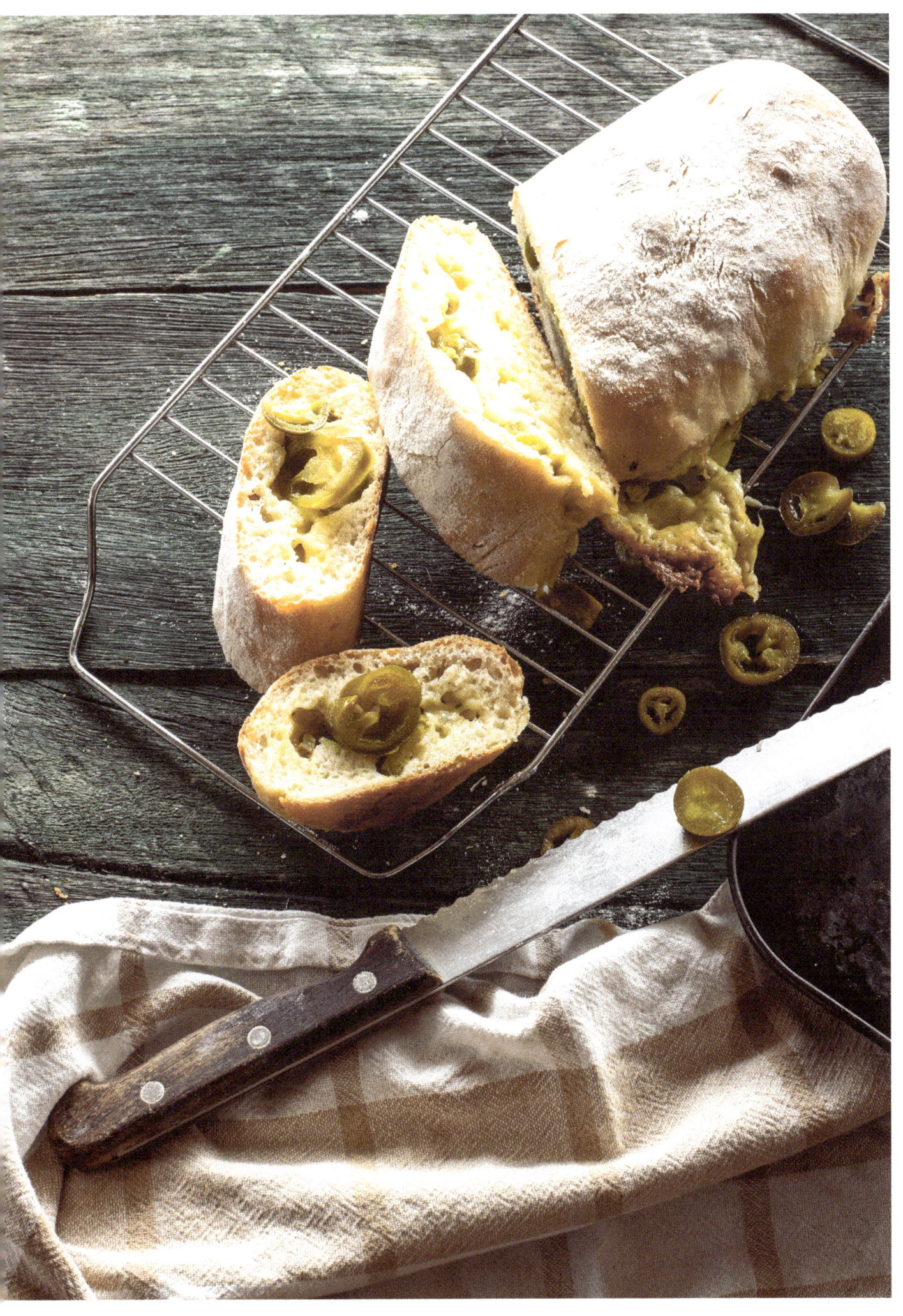

BREAM CREEK VINEYARD

Rabbit and Bream Creek Vineyard Pinot Noir

SERVES 4-6

This can also be cooked in the slow cooker for around 5 hours.

1 rabbit

plain flour to coat

extra virgin olive oil

12 shallots or baby brown onions

3 carrots

4 sticks celery

6 cloves garlic

4 bay leaves

6 sprigs thyme

pinch cracked black pepper

pinch sea salt

500ml Bream Creek Vineyard Pinot Noir

TO SERVE

creamy mashed potato or polenta

Heat the oven to 160°C.

Cut the rabbit into portions and roll each piece in flour. In a large heavy based pan with a dash of oil heated to medium high seal of the pieces of rabbit and transfer to a baking dish.

Peel the onions and add whole. Peel and dice the carrots into 2cm pieces. Chop the celery into 2cm pieces and add to the pan. Peel and crush the garlic. Add the bay leaf, thyme, pepper and pinot.

Cover the dish and cook for 2-3 hours until the rabbit is tender and falling off the bones.

Serve with creamy mashed potato or polenta and greens.

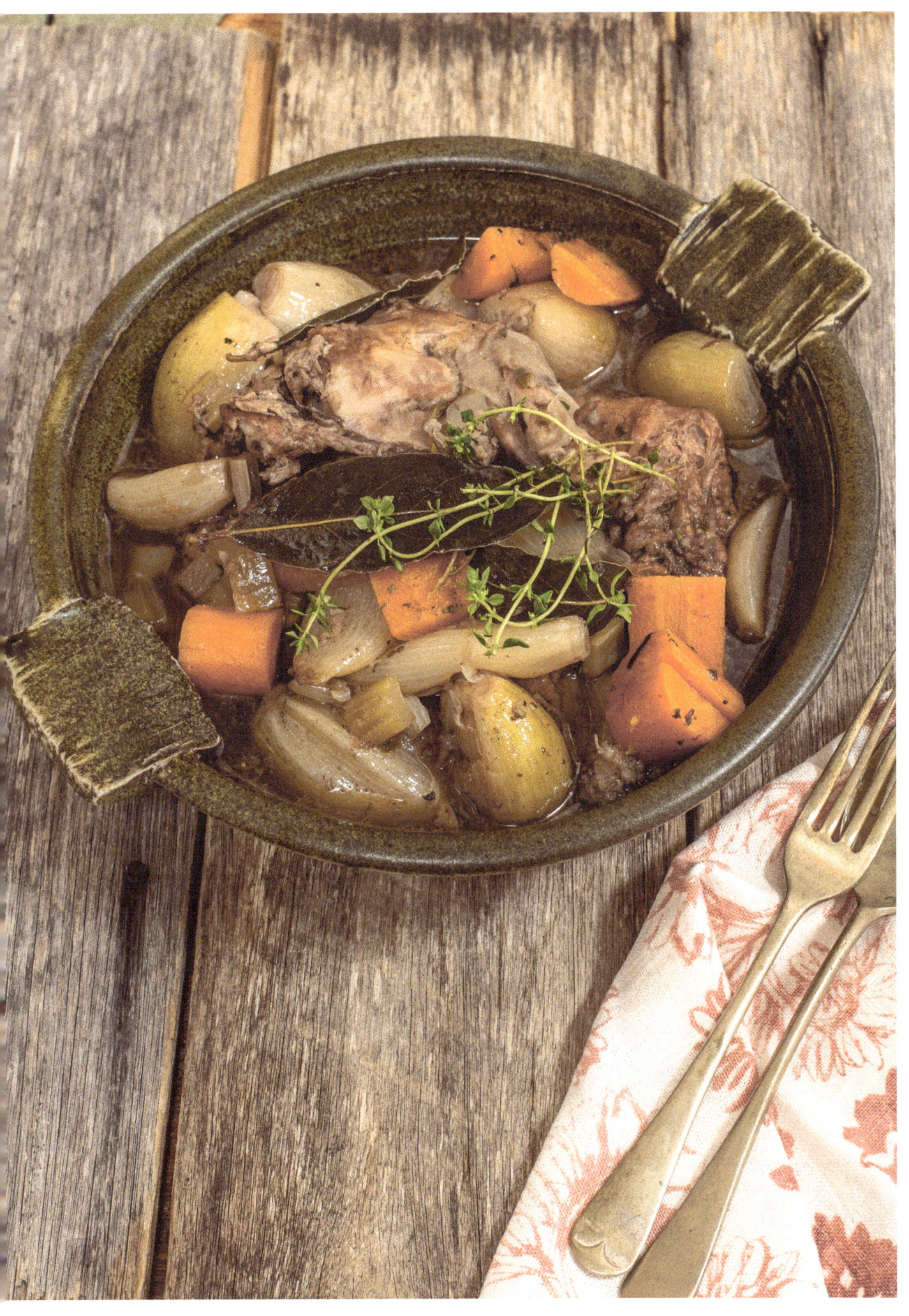

Pumpkin and Honey Gnocchi

SERVES 4-6

This easy way of making gnocchi - by boiling the potatoes it is different from the traditional method, and I find it a lot easier! If you are using good quality potatoes it works brilliantly and you'll find yourself making this gnocchi all the time. To save time, you can cook the gnocchi in advance and then reheat them in boiling water when it comes time to serve.

GNOCCHI

500 grams floury potatoes, such as Kennebec

2 eggs

½ teaspoon nutmeg

1 cup plain flour

salt

pepper

SAUCE

dash extra virgin olive oil

¼ pumpkin

2 brown onions

3 cloves garlic

2 cups mushrooms

20 sage leaves

½ bunch basil

2 tablespoons honey

2 cups spinach

80 grams parmesan to serve

To make the gnocchi, peel and dice the potatoes into 2cm cubes. Place potatoes in a saucepan, cover with water, bring to the boil and simmer for 18 minutes or until the potatoes are cooked through. Drain well and set aside to cool for a few minutes.

While the potatoes are still warm, mash well and stir through the eggs, nutmeg, flour and a pinch of salt and pepper. If the dough is too sticky to handle, add a little more flour. Using lightly floured hands, roll the dough into balls around the size of a ten cent piece, set aside on a lightly floured plate until ready to cook.

Heat the oven to 180°C.

Peel the pumpkin and dice in to around 1.5cm chunks and roast the pumpkin in a baking tray with a good splash of extra virgin olive oil for around 20 minutes until cooked.

To make the sauce, saute the finely sliced onion and crushed garlic in the extra virgin olive oil in a heavy based pan over a low heat. Add the mushrooms and continue sautéing until cooked through. Add the herbs and honey and hot gnocchi and toss through the spinach serve with the shaved parmesan.

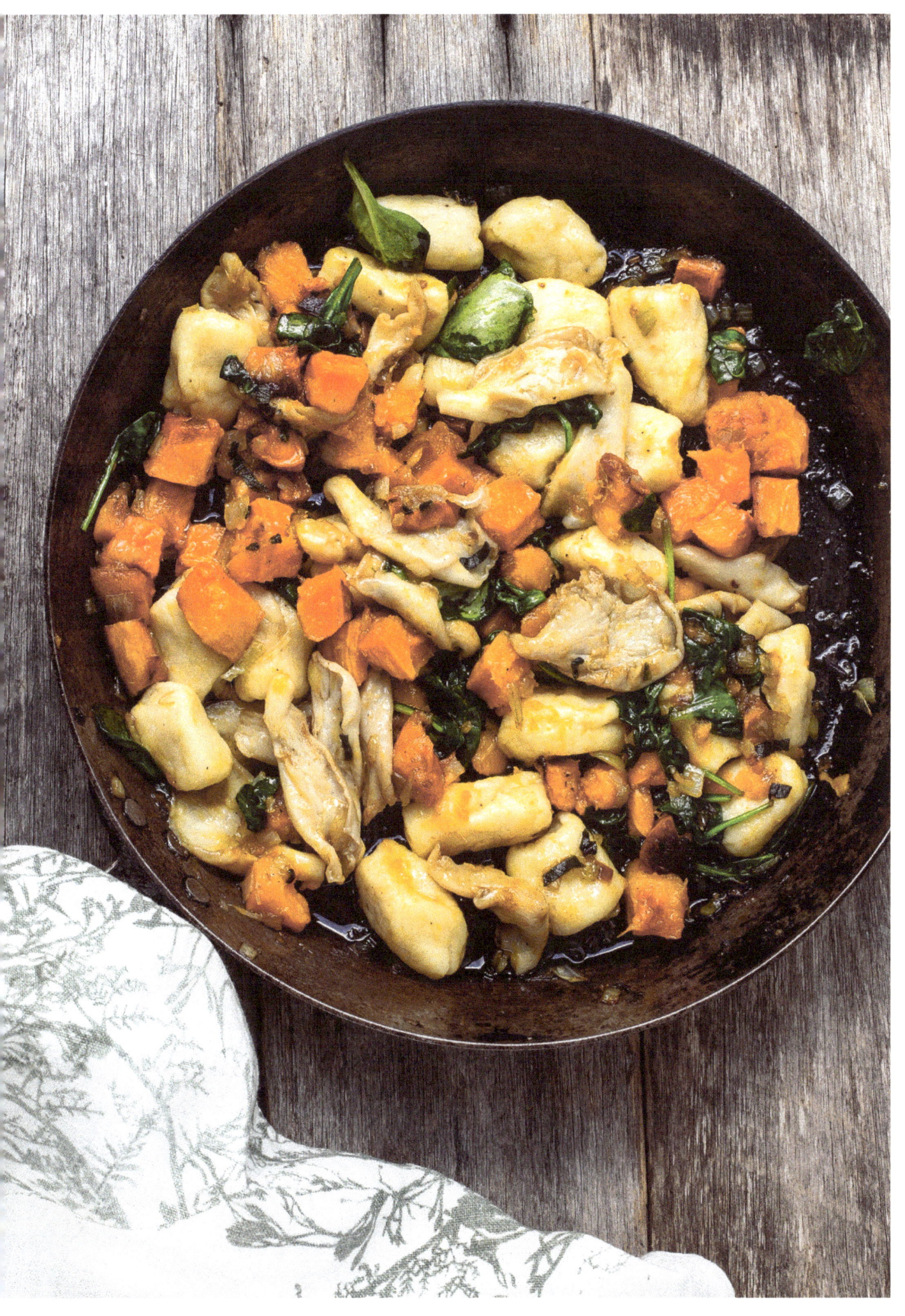

Tomato, Basil and Halloumi Salad

SERVES 4

Home grown in season tomatoes are the best, sharing my love of home grown tomatoes was my first post on my website back in 2012. There is at least a month where breakfast is simply tomatoes from the bowl ripening on the bench, on toast in our house each year. Pick a robust herbaceous peppery extra virgin olive oil and a good sprinkle of sea salt and that's flavour perfection there. Remember to save a few seeds from your best preforming tomatoes for the next year if you grow your own.. The seeds need to be fermented in a jar covered in cling film for a few days to remove the flesh and simply dried on newspaper. Apparently, there are thousands of varieties but mine end up being labeled are cherry (for salads and snacks), field (salads) and roma (for cooking), my garden is never organised or labeled very well and I've always forgotten the actual name by the time its time to harvest them. This simple salad is a meal on its own but would be lovely with chicken or lamb. I grow amazing basil, every tenth year or so...

200 grams haloumi or keflogravia cheese

plain flour for coating

robust extra virgin olive oil to cook and dress

lemon

salt

pepper

8 large field tomatoes

1 handful basil

sea salt

cracked pepper

Arrange your salad of sliced tomatoes and picked basil leaves on a beautiful platter and season well with salt, robust extra virgin olive oil and pepper.

To cook the haloumi, season the flour well with salt and pepper, heat a heavy based pan over a medium heat and heat the oil, dip each piece of cheese into the flour and then into the hot pan. We want crispy skinned cheese.

Place on the salad and drizzle with the robust oil and fresh squeezed lemon juice.

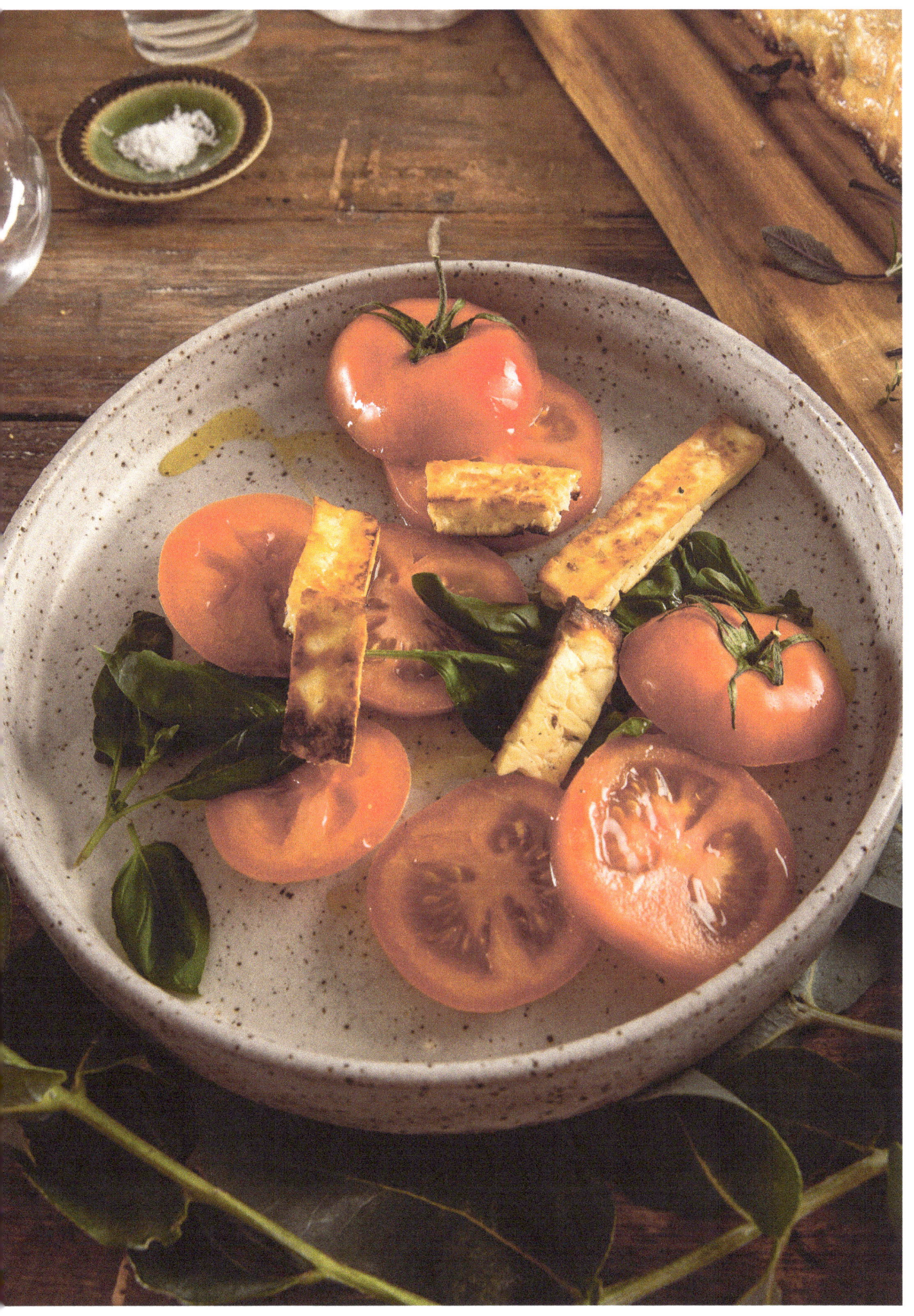

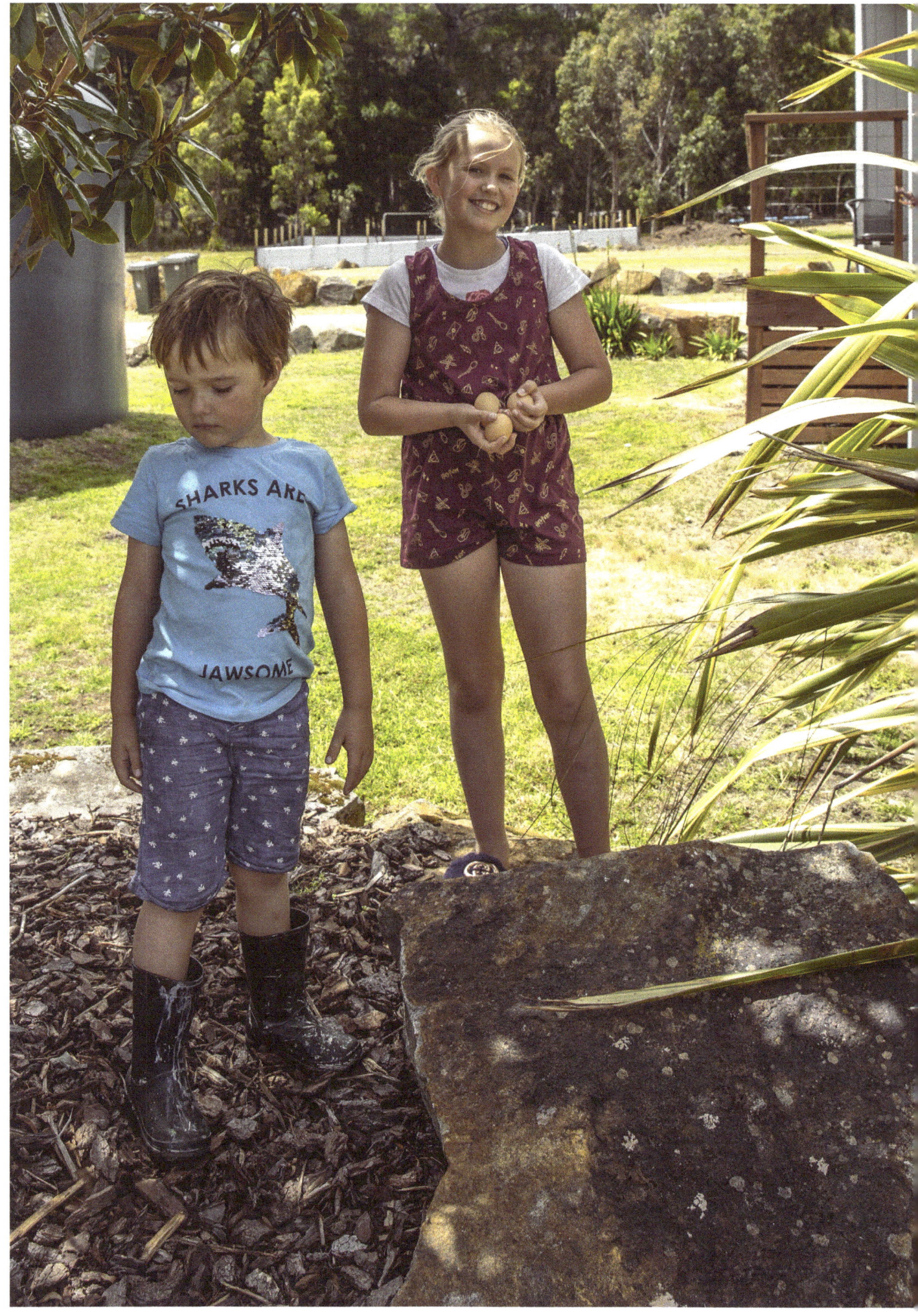

"Having chooks is great for kids. There's hours of entertainment searching for the egg stash. Freshly laid eggs cooked up for a lazy Sunday brunch...
what could be better?"

HILL STREET HOME

Lavender Granola

MAKES ONE BIG JAR ENOUGH FOR 12 OR MORE BREAKFASTS

This recipe is adapted from the crunchy muesli recipe in my first book The Real Food for Kids Cookbook. We make it all the time at home the kids can pick their own flavour combinations with the dried fruits and nuts they like. This version is a bit fancy with the addition of Imperial Gem culinary lavender from Campo De Flori and it is loved by our guests at Little Norfolk Bay Events and Chalets.

100ml delicate or medium extra virgin olive oil

3 tablespoons honey

4 cups rolled oats

½ cup desiccated coconut

½ cup almonds, slithered

2 teaspoons Campo De Flori Lavender

2 cups dried raisins

milk or yogurt to serve

Heat the oven to 170°C.

Mix together the oats, nuts and desiccated coconut. Warm the oil in a saucepan on the stove. Pour the syrup mixture into the oat mixture and mix well.

Divide the mixture on to 2 large baking dishes and bake, stirring every 5 minutes for 20 minutes until golden. Cool then stir through the dried fruit and lavender.

Serve with milk or yogurt for breakfast.

Dress up your breakfast table with beautiful tableware from Hill Street Home. We have used a unique vase to showcase the lavender for our spread.

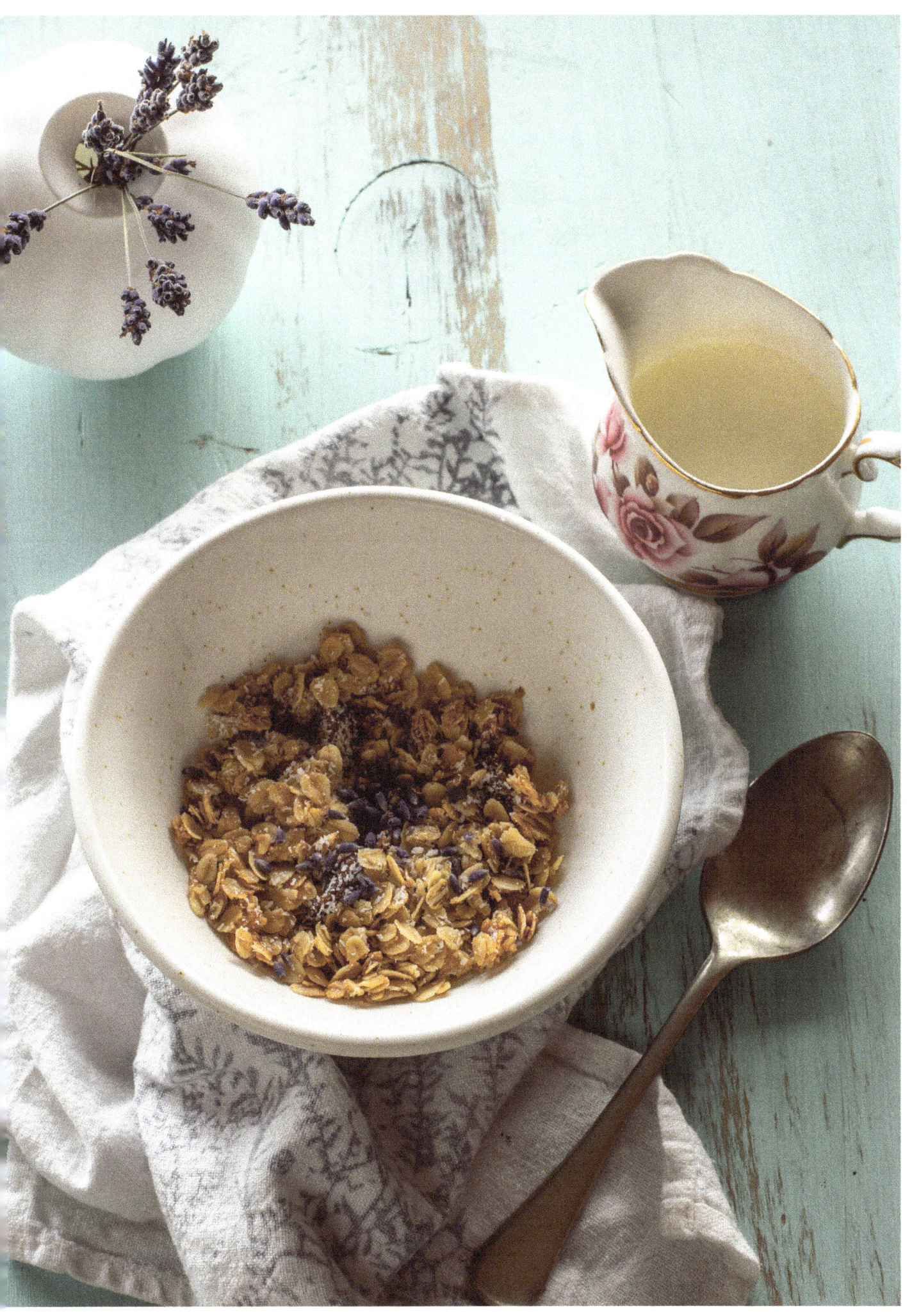

Radicchio, Green Olives, Parmesan and Honey

SERVES 4 AS A SIDE

Bitter radicchio and honey is a lovely combination with naturally fermented salty and bitter olives. A beautiful salad to accompany a rich roasted meat.

1 head radicchio

80 grams parmesan

100 grams olives

1 tablespoon honey

1 tablespoon red wine vinegar

2 tablespoons robust extra virgin olive oil

To make the dressing mix the honey, vinegar and oil together well.

Assemble the washed and spun radicchio leaves with the olives and shaved parmesan. Dress and serve immediately.

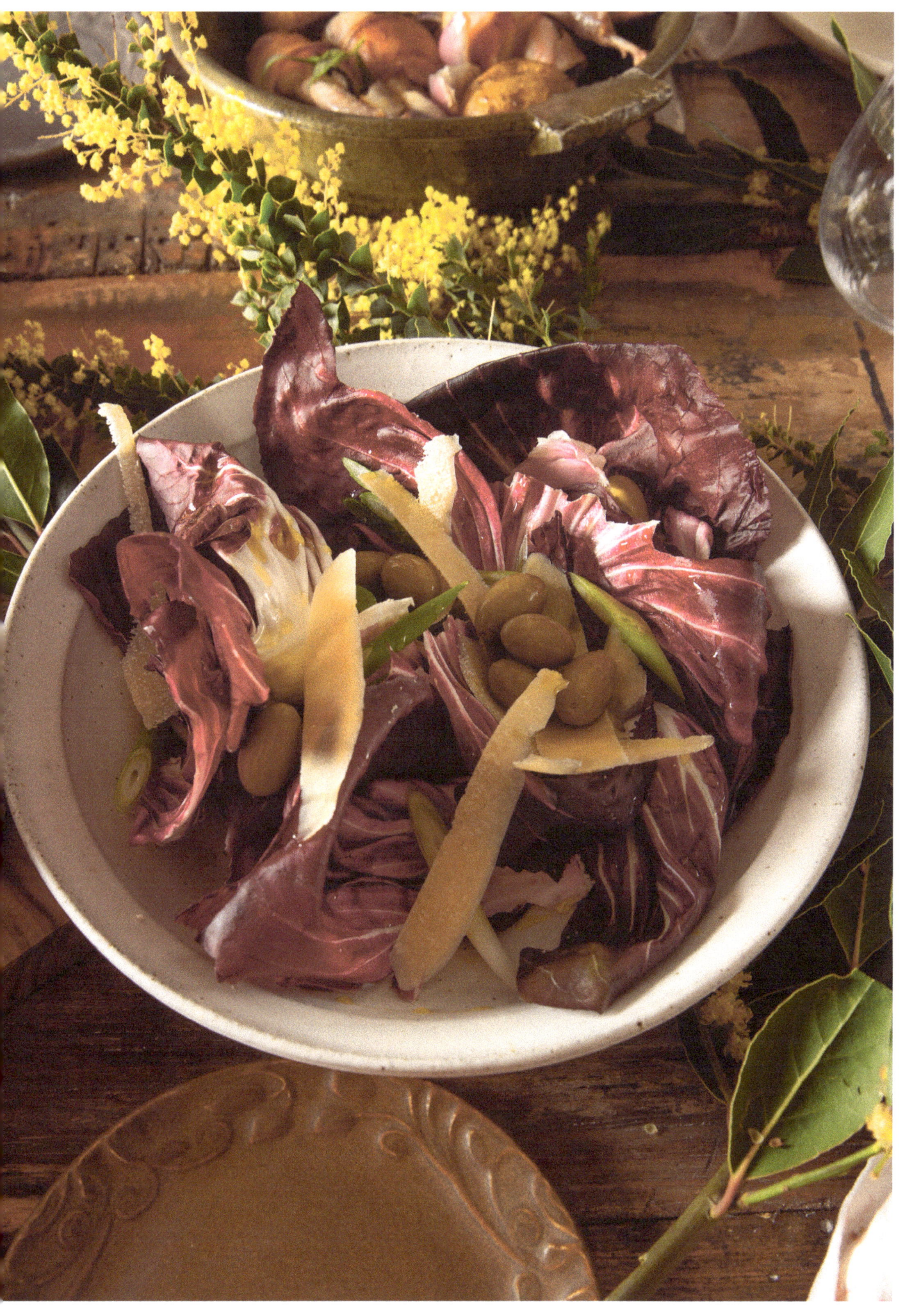

Pantry Hummus

SERVES 10

What is a home kitchen without hummus? For veggie sticks in the lunch box, to fill celery sticks with or on the spread for a special meal. This is a simplified recipe made a bit fancy finished sprinkled with Weston Farm's smoked paprika that you can smell the smokey smell from a few metres away. I make hummus with soaked and cooked chickpeas, soaked and cooked beans, tins of chickpeas or bean, frozen peas and even roast pumpkin and roast sweet potato. Probably nothing like an actual hummus.

200 grams cooked chickpeas

5 cloves garlic

approximately 100ml robust extra virgin olive oil

juice of 2 lemons

sea salt

pepper

1 teaspoon smoked paprika

In the thermocooker or blender blend all the ingredients together to form a smooth paste.

Season well with salt and pepper.

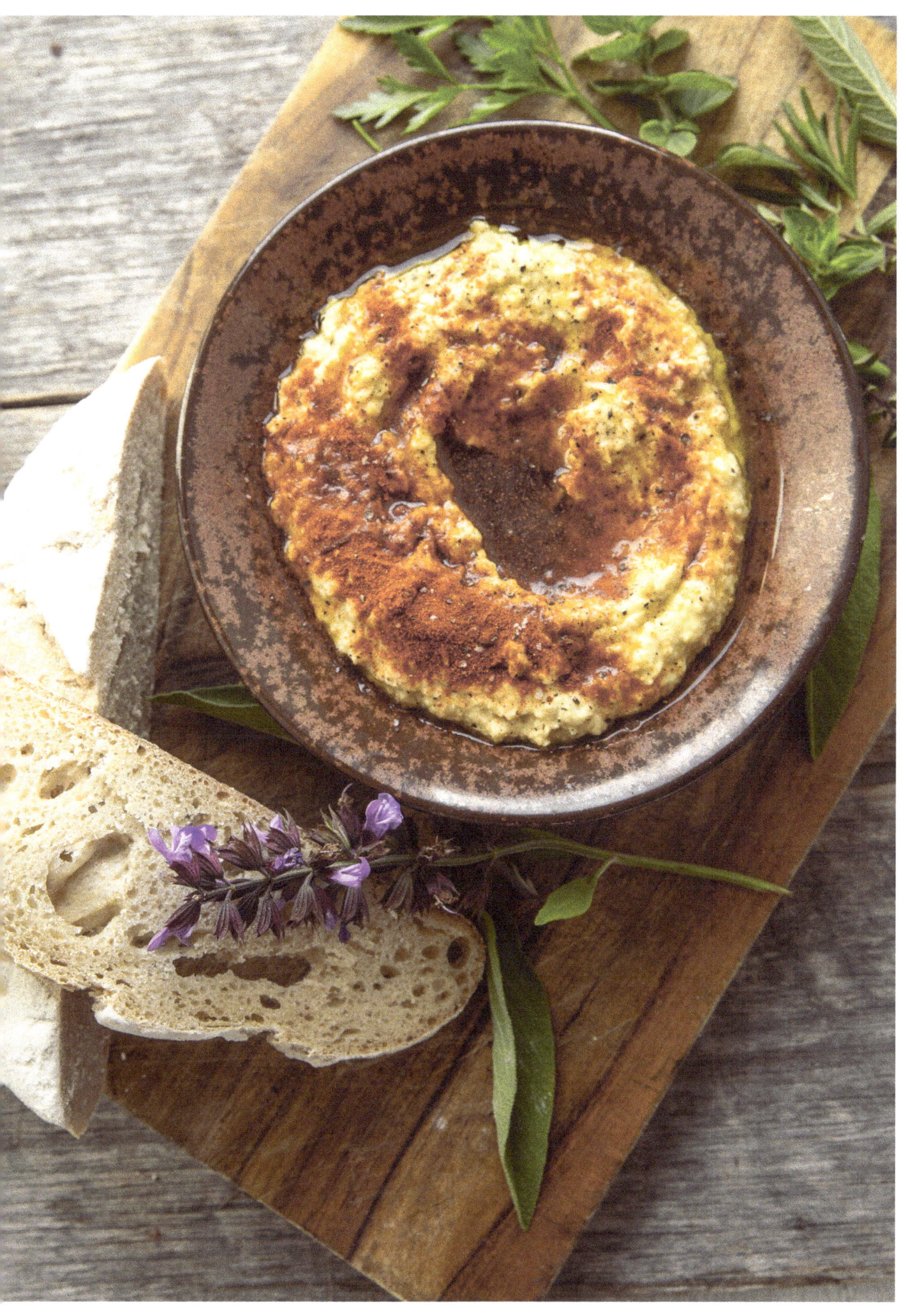

Venison Loin with Blue Cheese and Extra Virgin Olive Oil Risotto

SERVES 6

A risotto and a piece of meat on the barbeque is actually an easy way to prepare a fancy and impressive dinner.

600 grams venison loin

1100ml chicken or vegetable stock

1 tablespoon butter

1 onion

2 cloves garlic

350 grams arborio rice

100ml white wine

30 grams parmesan cheese

70 grams blue cheese

a few sprigs of parsley

2 cups spinach

100ml cream

100ml robust extra virgin olive oil

Bring the stock to a gentle boil in a saucepan.

Using another large, heavy-based saucepan, melt the butter over medium heat. Finely dice the onion and crush the garlic, add to the pan and sauté for 3 minutes, or until tender.

Add the rice and cook for one minute, stirring well. Add the wine and stir. Gradually add the hot stock, one ladleful at a time, stirring regularly – wait until each ladle of stock is almost fully absorbed by the rice before adding the next. This process will take 15-20 minutes.

Dice the blue cheese. Stir the cheese, cream and spinach through the risotto and add the parsley leaves. Cover and set aside to rest for a few minutes to finish cooking, and then serve immediately. If you have a thermocooker then you will know how to cook the risotto in it.

Leave the venison on the bench for at least one hour before cooking so that it is at room temperature. Heat a pan or the barbeque and cover the venison in oil cook over a medium high heat for a few minutes on each side. Venison is best served rare, it is low in fat so will be tough if over cooked.

Serve the venison with the risotto and season with salt and pepper and a good drizzle of the robust a peppery extra virgin olive oil.

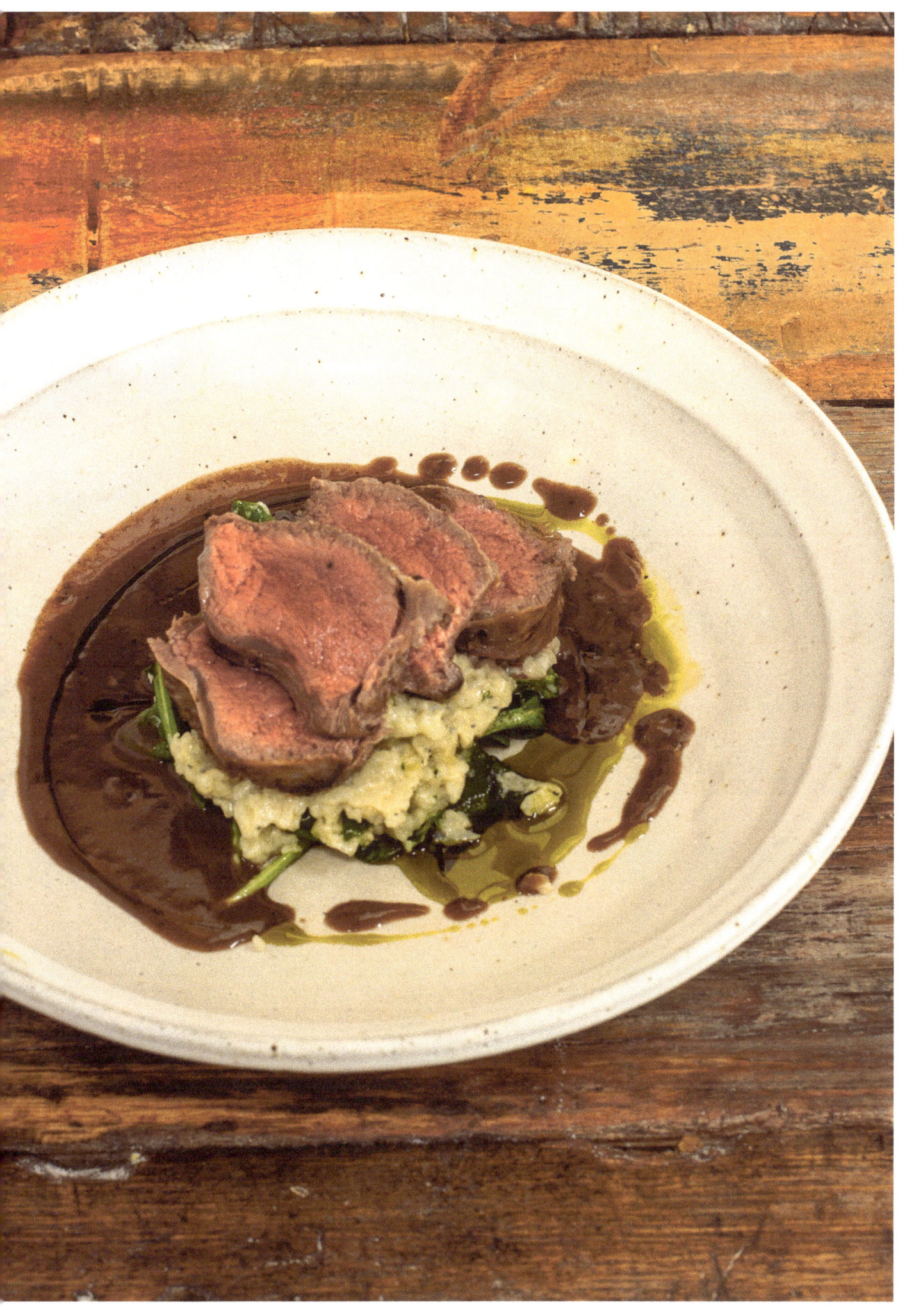

Parrot Fish, Lemon and Lavender En Papillote

SERVES 2

1 x 750 gram parrot fish, scaled and gutted

1 lemon

1 teaspoon culinary lavender

1 large pinch sea salt

pinch white pepper

delicate extra virgin olive oil

TO SERVE

a big salad dressed with extra virgin olive oil and lemon to serve with the fish

Heat the oven to 180°C.

Lay the gutted and scaled whole fish onto a large square of baking paper, I also use a large square of kitchen foil as well underneath the paper, to make sure the seal is tight when wrapping it up. Slice the lemon and lay on the fish and dump a few tablespoons of olive oil on top, sprinkle the lavender, sea salt and pepper over the fish and wrap up so that it is sealed tightly.

Place the wrapped fish on a baking tray and place the tray into the oven. Depending on the fat content of your fish, the size of the fish and your oven, the cooking time will vary, but check after 10 minutes and then continue to cook until it is just cooked through or slightly under.

To check if the fish is cooked the fin should slip out easily or just check to see if the flesh is flaking of the bone.

Serve immediately as it will continue cooking.

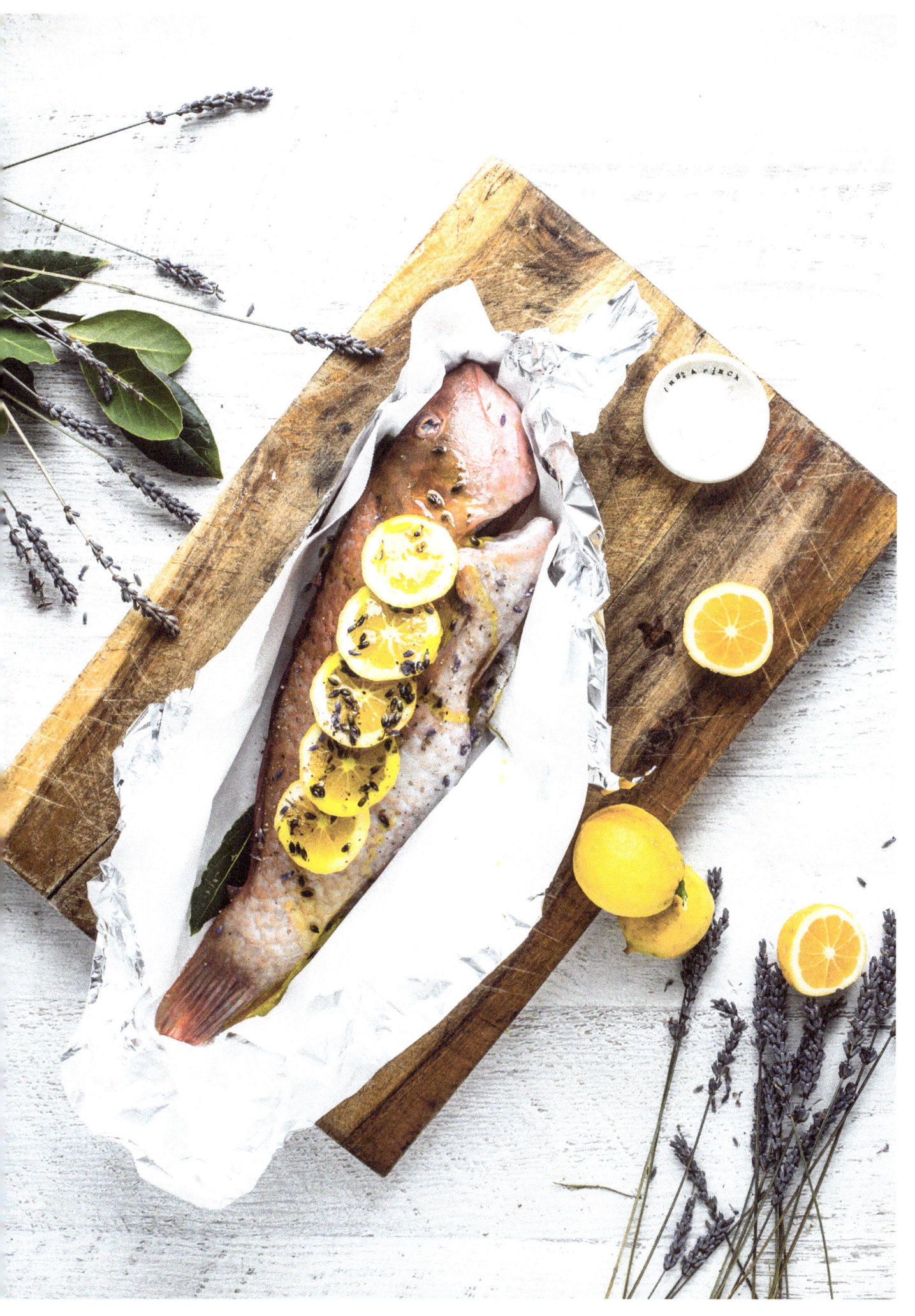

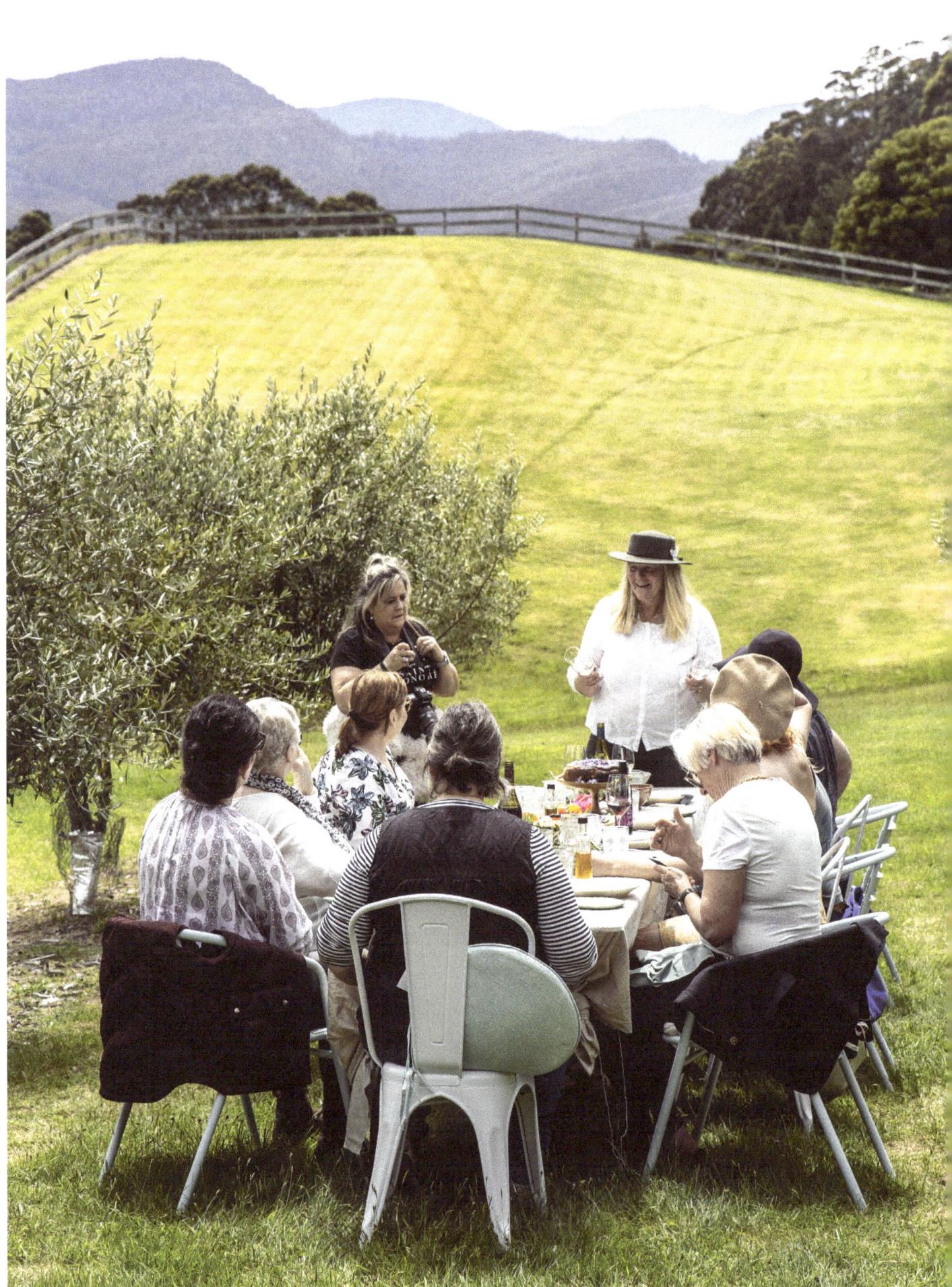

"There is nothing better than good food shared with great people."

French Onion Soup

SERVES 8

Making your own stock makes the best tasting soups and sauces. I find using the slow cooker the simplest way to make small batches of stock at home from the bones I get with my Summerlea Farm Beef box.

STOCK

1 kilo beef bones

3 sprigs thyme

2 bay leaves

pepper

salt

1 leek

2 carrots

2 brown onions

2 sticks celery

(or trimmings from carrots, leek, celery, onion and tomatoes you have collected while cooking and frozen).

SOUP

1 kilo brown onions

1 teaspoon butter

2 tablespoons brown sugar

Heat the oven to 160°C.

Trim the fat from the bones and bake them in the oven to brown in a baking tray for 20 minutes. Put them in the slow cooker with the thyme, bay leaf, onion ends, pinch of salt and pepper, vegetables or trimmings and 2 litres of water, cook on high for 8 hours. Strain and refrigerate the stock so the fat settles on top, discard the fat.

Slice the onions and fry in hot pot for 5 minutes, making sure they get some colour, add the sugar and cook for a few minutes until the sugar caramelises. Add the stock and continue to cook for a further 15 minutes.

Season with salt and pepper and serve.

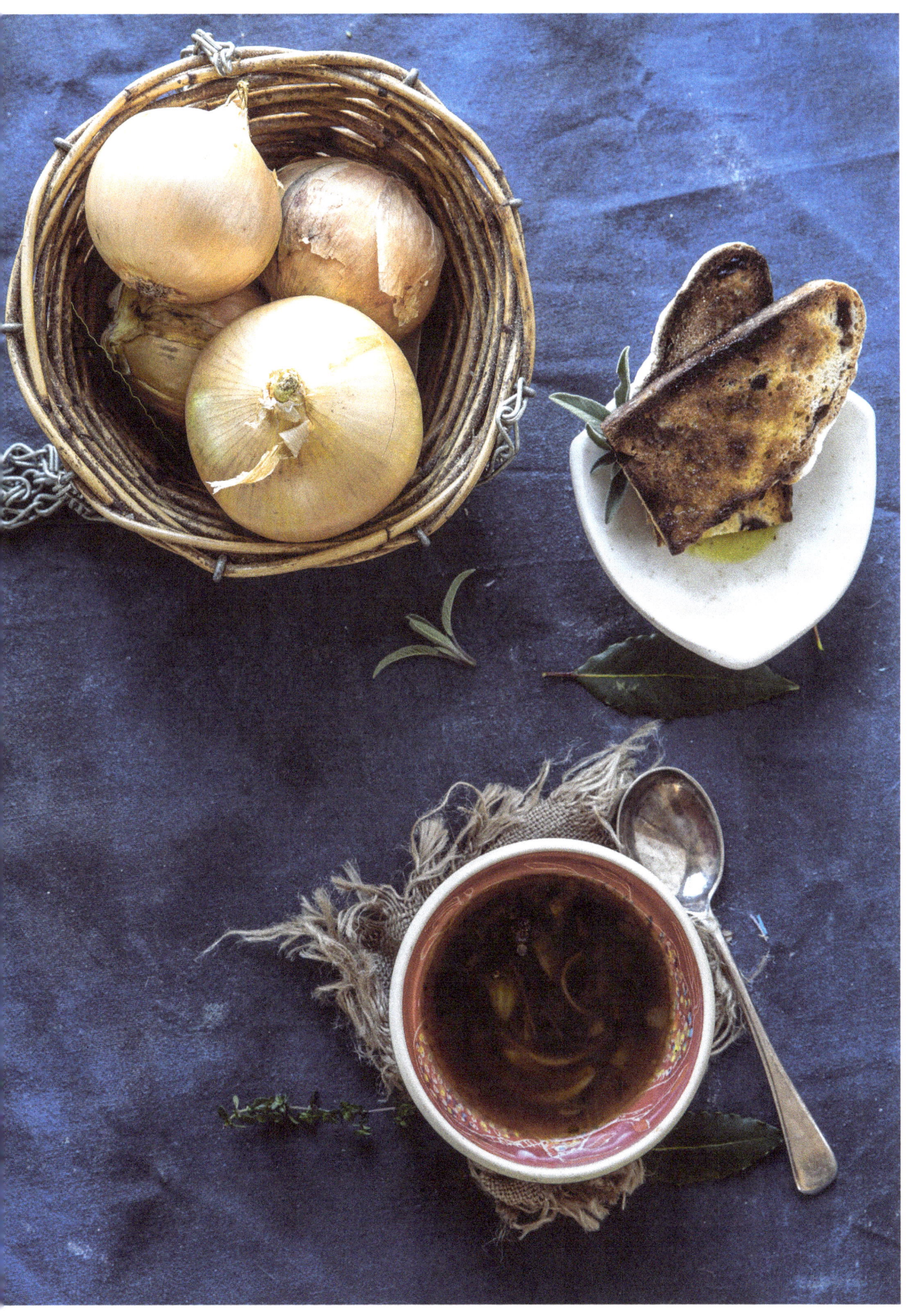

Mures Blue Eye Tartare

SERVES 4

Recipe by Markella Koutalidi, Mures Upper Deck

FOR TARTARE

300 grams Blue Eye Trevalla (skinless)

40 grams chopped pickled ginger

6 grams chopped curly leaf parsley

2 grams chopped dill

salt flakes

extra virgin olive oil

FOR GREEN GAZPACHO

250 grams cherry tomatoes

100 grams spinach leaves

100 grams curly leaf parsley

200ml of water

1 small cucumber (seeded and skinned)

1 small green capsicum (seeded)

15 grams brown onion

½ clove garlic

15ml white wine vinegar

tobasco

salt flakes

pepper

extra virgin olive oil

FOR GARNISH

80 grams wakame salad

20 grams of sesame seeds

3-4 baby radishes

optional: edible flowers such as Sorrel and Nasturtium

For the Gazpacho, create a tomato water: Blend cherry tomatoes on a high speed until smooth consistency is achieved. Place blended tomatoes in a pot and bring to the boil, then strain tomatoes through an oil filter. This makes roughly 100ml of tomato water. Cool in the fridge.

Create chlorophyll water: Blend spinach leaves, parsley and 200ml of water until a smooth consistency is achieved. Strain with a sieve, to achieve chlorophyll water. Cool in the fridge. Add tomato water, cucumber, capsicum, onion, garlic, white wine vinegar and a few drops of the chlorophyll water into a blender. Add a drizzle of olive oil and blend on high speed for four minutes. Season to taste with tobasco, salt and pepper.

For the Blue Eye Tartare, remove the skin and clean the fillets from the bloodline before finely dice your fish fillets. Place them in a bowl with the pickled ginger, parsley and dill, then add a generous sprinkling of salt flakes and a drizzle of olive oil. Mix thoroughly in bowl and adjust to your taste.

Toast sesame seeds at 120°C for 4 minutes. Thinly slice baby radishes. Place a biscuit cutting ring on the serving plate and fill with the tartare mixture. Press down lightly. Remove ring and drizzle gazpacho around the base of the tartare. Layer the top of the tartare with baby radish then the wakame salad and sprinkle dish with toasted sesame seeds.

For additional garnish you can add edible flowers such as sorrel and nasturtium from the garden.

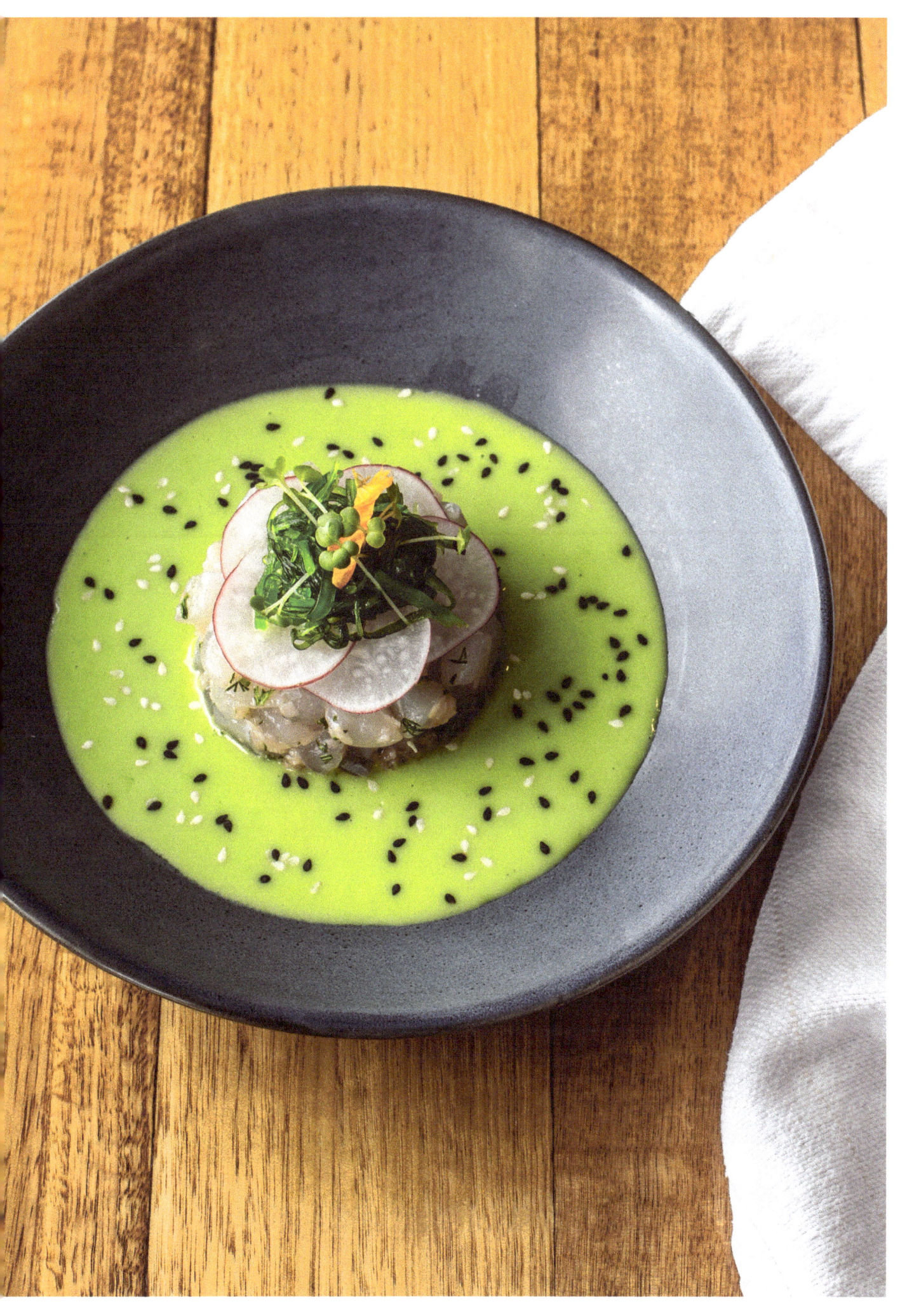

INDEX

A
Abalone Confit 124

Apple Cinnamon and Honey Porridge 110

B
Baked Beans 114

Baked Quince and Blue Cheese and Vino Cotta 52

Beef Marinated in Wild Pepper Isle's Tasmanian Pepper Berry Soy served with a Thai Noodle Salad 130

Beer Battered Scallops with Tartare Sauce 100

Beetroot Wellington 58

Blue Cheese Arancini 64

Blue Warhou Tartare 50

C
Cabbage Rolls 54

Campo De Flori Lavender Aioli with Crayfish Bruschetta 28

Chicken and Corn Soup 118

Chicken Liver Pate 126

Chicken Minestrone 120

Chorizo, Chilli, Freycinet Marine Farm Mussels and Handmade Pasta 74

Crayfish Bisque 10

Croissants 48

D
Duck Confit served with Puddleduck Vineyard Pinot Noir Jam and Slaw 94

F
French Onion Soup 166

Frozen Van Diemans Land Creamery Salted Caramel Tiramisu 22

Fruit Loaf 14

G
Garlic and Herb Pull Apart 106

Garlic, Feta and Herb Pizza 108

Goats Cheese Ravioli with Brown Butter and Sage 96

Green Tomato and Lentil Soup 12

H
Hazelnut and Green Peppercorn Crusted Lamb with Lost Pipin Cider and Apple Risotto 72

Hot and Sour Wakame and Cameron of Tasmania Oysters Broth 62

INDEX

J
Jalapeño Bread 144

L
Lamb Kashmir Korma 136
Lavender Granola 154
Leek and Apple Soup with Freshfield Grove Lemon Agrumato 88
Lenah Game Meats Wallaby Fillet with Goats Cheese and Cherry Chutney 60

M
Meander Valley Dairy Scones 102
Mures Blue Eye Tartare 168

O
Octopus Baked with Tomato, Olives and Jalapenos 84
Overnight Oat Ideas 112
Oysters with Lemon Agrumato and Pickled Fennel 90

P
Pantry Hummus 158
Parrot Fish Hong Kong Style 36
Parrot Fish, Lemon and Lavender En Papillote 162
Pickled Octopus 134
Pork Belly, Apple and Fennel cooked in Bream Creek Vineyard Sauvignon Blanc 86
Pumpkin and Honey Gnocchi 148

Q
Quail Roasted with Bacon and Tarragon with Garlic Roast Pink Eyes and Green Beans 66
Quail with a Quinoa, Citrus and Herb Salad 16
Quince, Lavender and Freshfield Grove Extra Virgin Olive Oil Cake 70

R
Rabbit and Bream Creek Vineyard Pinot Noir 146
Radicchio, Green Olives, Parmesan and Honey Salad 156
Raw Striped Trumpeter Kohlrabi Quick Pickle 30
Rhubard Cream Brulee 132

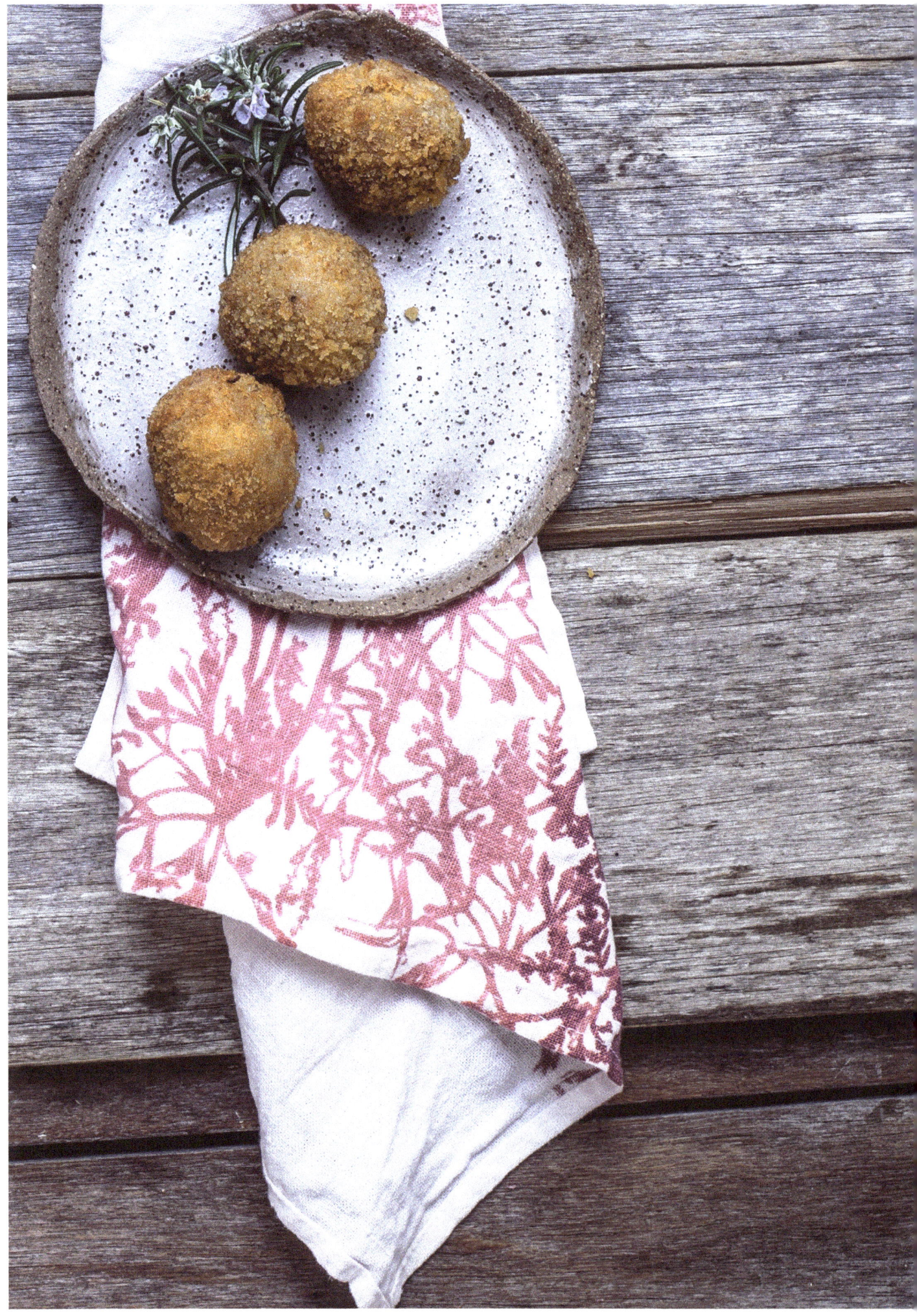

INDEX

S
Salmon and Saffron Butter 38
Salmon Carpaccio 138
Sautéed Lentil Stuffed Tomato 78
Scallops and Handmade Pasta 98
Smoked Oyster Pate 122
Sourdough 40
Spiced Cauliflower and Labneh 76
Striped Trumpeter Confit 34
Summerlea Farm Flat Iron Steak Marinated in Preserved Lemon, Green Pepper and Horseradish ... 24

T
Taramasalata 142
Tassal Hot Smoked Salmon, Blue Cheese, Rocket and Apple Salad with a Honey and Mustard Dressing ... 18
Tomato, Basil and Halloumi Salad 150

V
Venison Loin with Blue Cheese and Extra Virgin Olive Oil Risotto 160

W
Wallaby Shanks Braised with Paprika 82

Z
Zucchini and Tomato Stew 26

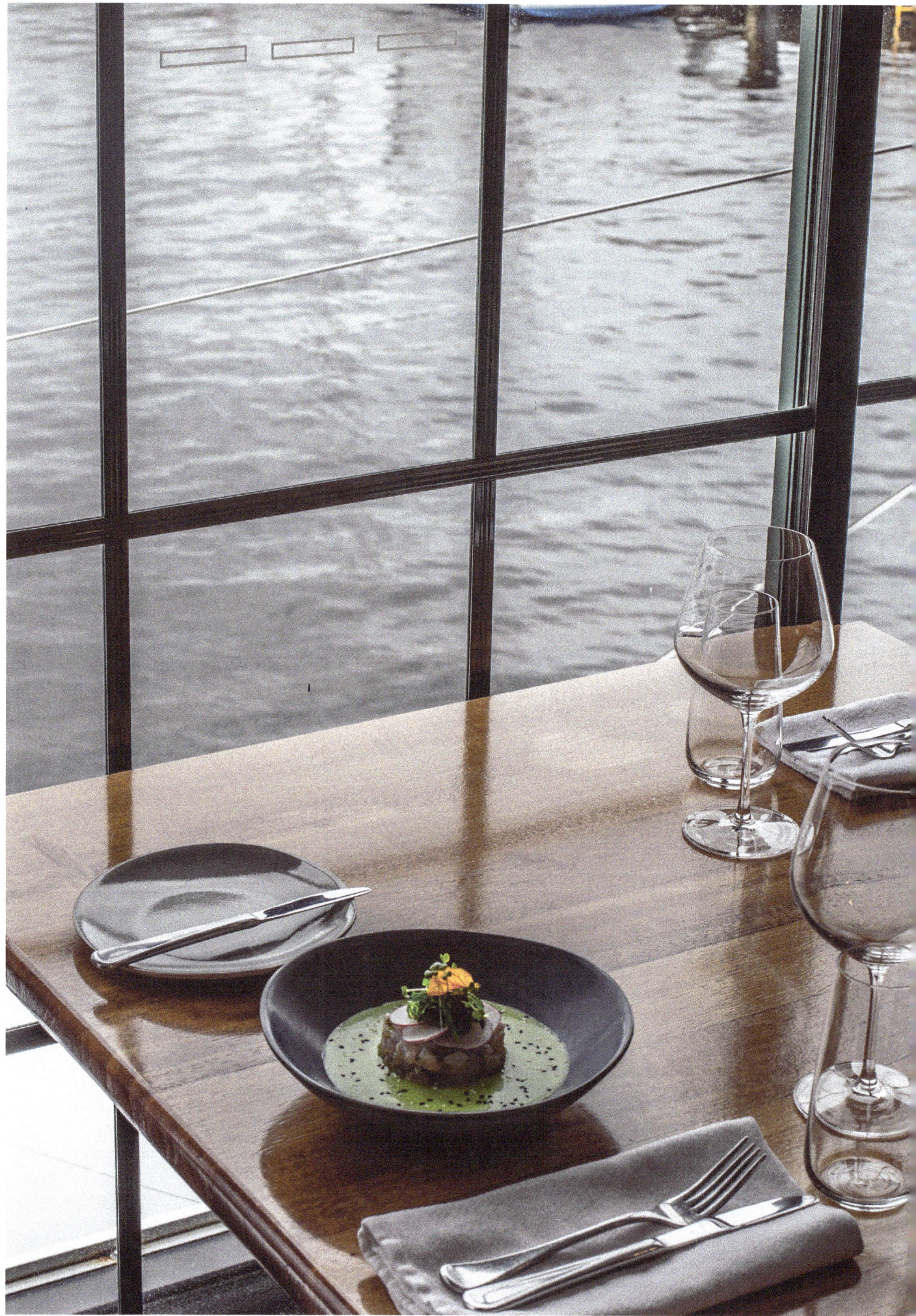

"I try to support local businesses. One thing 2020 has taught us, is that its pretty inconvenient when the things you need aren't grown or produced in your state."

THANK YOU TO OUR GENEROUS SPONSORS

EST. 1974

Bream Creek Vineyard

◊ TASMANIA ◊

BREAM CREEK VINEYARD

Bream Creek Vineyard is one of the pioneers of the modern Tasmanian wine industry. The vineyard was planted in 1974, making it amongst the earliest commercial vineyards established in Tasmania and was purchased in 1990 by Fred Peacock, one of Tasmania's leading viticulturists. We produce a wide range of award-winning wines, so we are confident we will have a wine to suit your tastes. Beginning with traditional method sparkling wines, moving through a wide range of white wines and a Pinot Noir rosé, two different styles of Pinot Noir, a Cabernet Merlot and finishing with a delicious lighter styled late picked dessert wine. We have a cellar door opening in August 2020 at the top of the vineyard with amazing views down to Marion Bay and Maria Island and look forward to welcoming you for a tutored tasting of our wines!

0419 363 714
fred@breamcreekvineyard.com.au
www.breamcreekvineyard.com.au

THANK YOU TO OUR GENEROUS SPONSORS

CAMERON OF TASMANIA

Located on the pristine South-East Coast of Tasmania, Cameron of Tasmania is a dynamic family business working for over 30 years as a vertically integrated oyster company. Camerons supplies world class oyster products, ranging from spat to large oysters, Australia wide and to selected overseas destinations.

03 6253 5111
admin@cameronsoysters.com
www.cameronsoysters.com

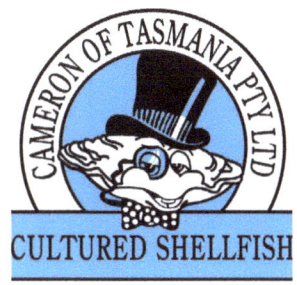

CAMPO DE FLORI

Discover a world of beauty at Campo de Flori. There's only one place in the world like Campo de Flori, where a whole world of beautiful tastes, views and experiences can be had in the one place. We are the only farm in Tasmania offering farm tours of saffron, lavender, olives with a cellar door for tasting and a ceramics studio where we can offer a true paddock to 'made here' plate on a farm.

Discover ceramics classes, take a farm visit, learn all about lavender, taste the beauty of the extra virgin olive oil and buy award winning saffron and culinary lavender from the farm gate. Located in beautiful Glen Huon, Campo de Flori is waiting for you to visit.

03 6266 6370
lisa@campodeflori.com.au
www.campodeflori.com

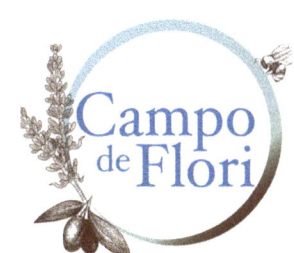

CHRISTMAS HILL RASPBERRY FARM

Located just off the Bass Highway between Elizabeth Town and Deloraine, Christmas Hills Raspberry Farm was established in 1984 when the Dornauf family planted twelve acres of raspberry canes on a north facing hill on their property.

In 1995 the café was built and is now a dining hotspot for locals and tourists alike.

In December 2012 the new shop was opened creating more space for customers to enjoy all the deliciousness the Raspberry Farm Cafe has to offer

03 6362 2186
info@raspberryfarmcafe.com
9 Christmas Hills Rd, Elizabeth Town Tasmania
raspberryfarmcafe.com

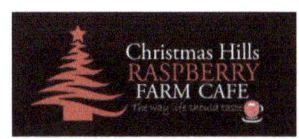

THANK YOU TO OUR GENEROUS SPONSORS

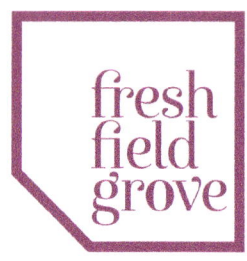

FRESHFIELD GROVE

Fiona and Glenn have a 1000 tree olive grove in the Coal River Valley. There is evidence that olive oil has been produced by humans for thousands of years, but at Freshfield Grove they use a modern Italian press to produce their small batch cold pressed extra virgin olive oil. The cool climate and low rainfall leads to fruit that ripens slowly and is full of complex flavours. Their oil packs a real punch, which means that a little goes a long way, and it can be used to add an intense splash of Tasmanian flavour to a wide variety of dishes.

0400 127 447
farmerfi@freshfieldgrove.com.au
49 Tea Tree Road, Campania, Tasmania
www.freshfieldgrove.com.au

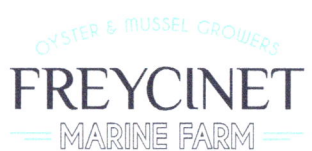

FREYCINET MARINE FARM

Bringing the pristine tastes and stories of the unique seas of Tasmania to life. Taste some of Tasmania's best fresh seafood – enjoyed fresh on our deck or taken away. Oysters and mussels harvested fresh from our farm daily, scallops, abalone and rocklobster, salmon sourced from local fisherman.

Our daily farm tours are now available in an exciting new format, our partner business, Oyster Bay Tours, is now offering water and land based walking tours of the farm.

03 6257 0261
oysters@freycinetmarinefarm.com
1784 Coles Bay Rd, Coles Bay, Tasmania
oysterbaytours.com

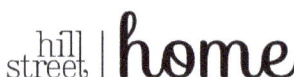

HILL STREET HOME

Located within our Devonport, Sandy Bay and West Hobart stores, Hill Street Home features a carefully curated collection of beautiful flowers, gifts, hand-made chocolates and gift hampers.

We deliver Australia-wide.

03 6234 6849
home.hillstreetgrocer.com

LENAH GAME MEATS

Lenah Game Meats was established in 1993 with the primary purpose of bringing Lenah Wallaby to the world. It's a uniquely Tasmanian meat, wild harvested from grasslands producing a mild sweet tasting meat. Lenah Wallaby is harvested using deep ethical principles in balance with our environment. Lenah is a Tasmanian Aboriginal word for wallaby.

03 6326 1777
admin@lenah.com.au
www.lenah.com.au

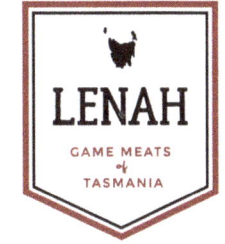

LOST PIPPIN

Real Cider - Cider from apples, perry from pears, styles not flavours
Real Fruit - 100% Tasmanian apples and pears
Real People - Proudly independent and owner operated since 2012

0417 569 163
Cranston, Richmond, Tasmania
lostpippin.com.au

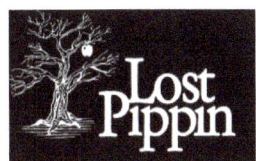

PUDDLEDUCK VINEYARD PINOT NOIR

Grown on site using Darren's favourite clones and low yields, our pinot noir is a lush fruit driven example of what the Coal River Valley can produce. Lots of black cherry and raspberry on the nose with hints of black currant and pepper on the palate, and super rich silky tannins to finish. Our pinot noir will only get better with time, with its best drinking in five to eight years' time. Fantastic with lamb, game meats, dishes with mushrooms or truffles and of course duck.

Try our "Reverse BYO®" picnics: You supply the picnic food - we supply the beverages!

03 6260 2301
www.puddleduck.com.au
992 Richmond Road, Richmond, Tasmania

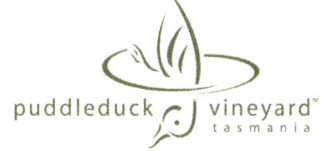

THANK YOU TO OUR GENEROUS SPONSORS

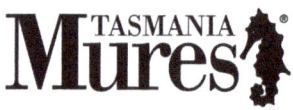

MURES TASMANIA

Jill & George Mure established Mures Fish House in 1973 in Battery Point, Hobart. When they struggled to source quality, fresh, local seafood, George went fishing.

More than 40 years on, now owned by Will & Judy Mure, Mures Tasmania remains a vertically integrated Tasmanian business from hook to plate that still loves quality, fresh, local seafood.

Victoria Dock, Hobart Tasmania
243 Kennedy Drive, Cambridge Tasmania
www.mures.com.au

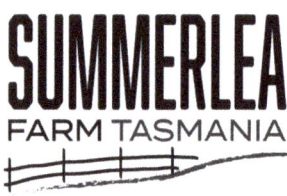

SUMMERLEA FARM

Summerlea Farm in North Lilydale is entirely family owned and operated. Rick and Liz produce 100% grass fed, single origin beef. All beef sold comes exclusively from their property – born and raised quietly as part of a small herd on their farm. Seasonal Beef Boxes are sold via subscription and direct to customer online. They are carefully curated to ensure each box includes a variety of cuts prepared in a number of ways. Their beef has featured on menus at the award winning Agrarian Kitchen Eatery and Dark Mofo's Winter Feast. You'll also find a selection of Summerlea Farm beef cuts expertly butchered at Bayside Meats in Sandy Bay.

Lilydale, Tasmania 7268
summerleafarmtas@outlook.com
summerleafarmtasmania.com

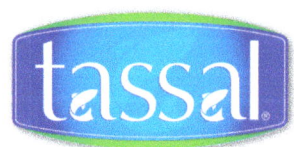

TASSAL

Our Home is Tasmania, a beautiful island with cool waters and a rich maritime history where our ambition to produce healthy, fresh Atlantic salmon began more than 30 years ago. From humble beginnings, we are Australia's largest producer of Tasmanian grown Atlantic salmon, our focus on quality and sustainability has underpinned our reputation as a global pioneer and leader. The management of food quality is of critical importance and we have extensive policies and procedures in place aimed at the consistent production of high quality, safe food for all consumers.

03 6244 9025
Tassal Salmon Shop, 2 Salamanca Square, Hobart Tasmania
www.tassal.com.au

THANK YOU TO OUR GENEROUS SPONSORS

TASFOODS LTD

TasFoods is the Tasmanian food specialist. We are the trusted source for premium Tasmanian products fit for the world stage. Our products are the essence of Tasmania.

TasFoods is a diversified food business focussed on leveraging the natural attributes of Tasmania's agricultural & food production environment to create premium food products for sale to Australian & export consumers.

61 3 6331 6983
admin@tasfoods.com.au
54 Tamar St, Launceston Tasmania 7250
www.tasfoods.com.au

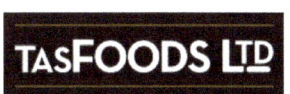

VAN DIEMENS LAND CREAMERY

Established in 2005, Van Diemens Land Creamery was created by a Tasmanian Dairy farming family. Today, Van Diemens Land Creamery's product can be found in premium restaurants, delicatessens and scoop outlets right around Tasmania, Victoria, NSW and WA. They continue to proudly use fresh, local produce to make premium, authentic ice cream, so you can experience the essence of Tasmania.

0448 849 724
hobart@vdlcreamery.com.au
Constitution Dock, Hobart Tasmania
www.vdlcreamery.com.au

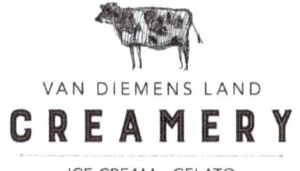

WILD PEPPER ISLE

Wild Pepper Isle is a vertically integrated bushfood business based in Hobart. They sustainable harvest native Tasmanian native bushfood such as Tasmanian Pepperberry and kunzea ambigua and hand-make award winning bushfood products.

Their ethos is to build a connection to the land through sustainably harvested native bushfood and to bring those fantastic flavours to households across Australia.

0457 531 559
info@wildpepperisle.com.au
www.wildpepperisle.com.au

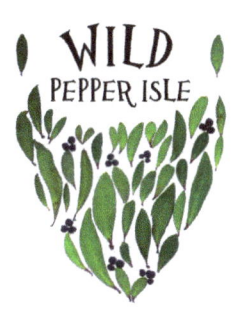

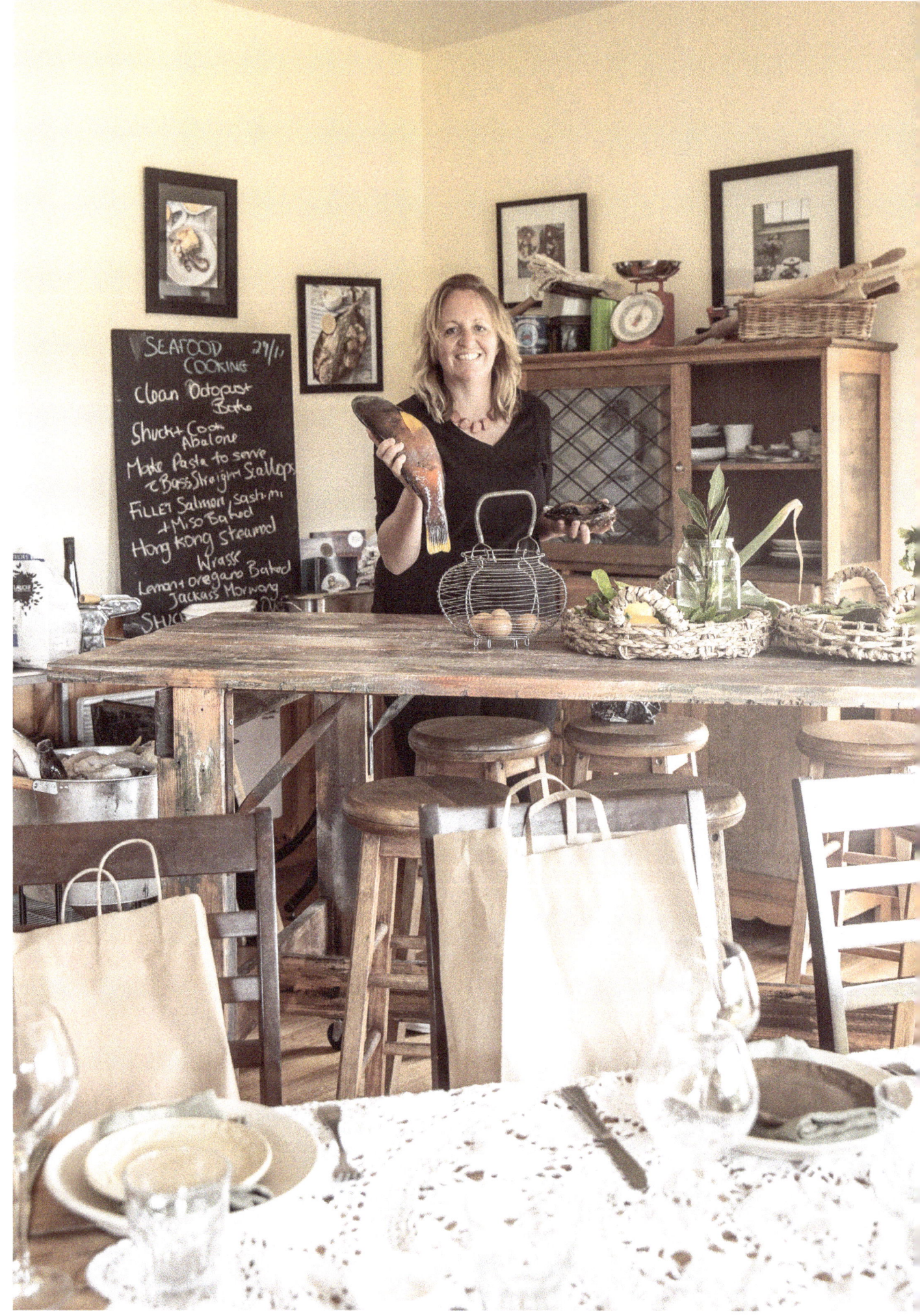

"I hope I have inspired you to get into the kitchen and enjoy feeding your family and friends, and most of all...yourself. You deserve it!"

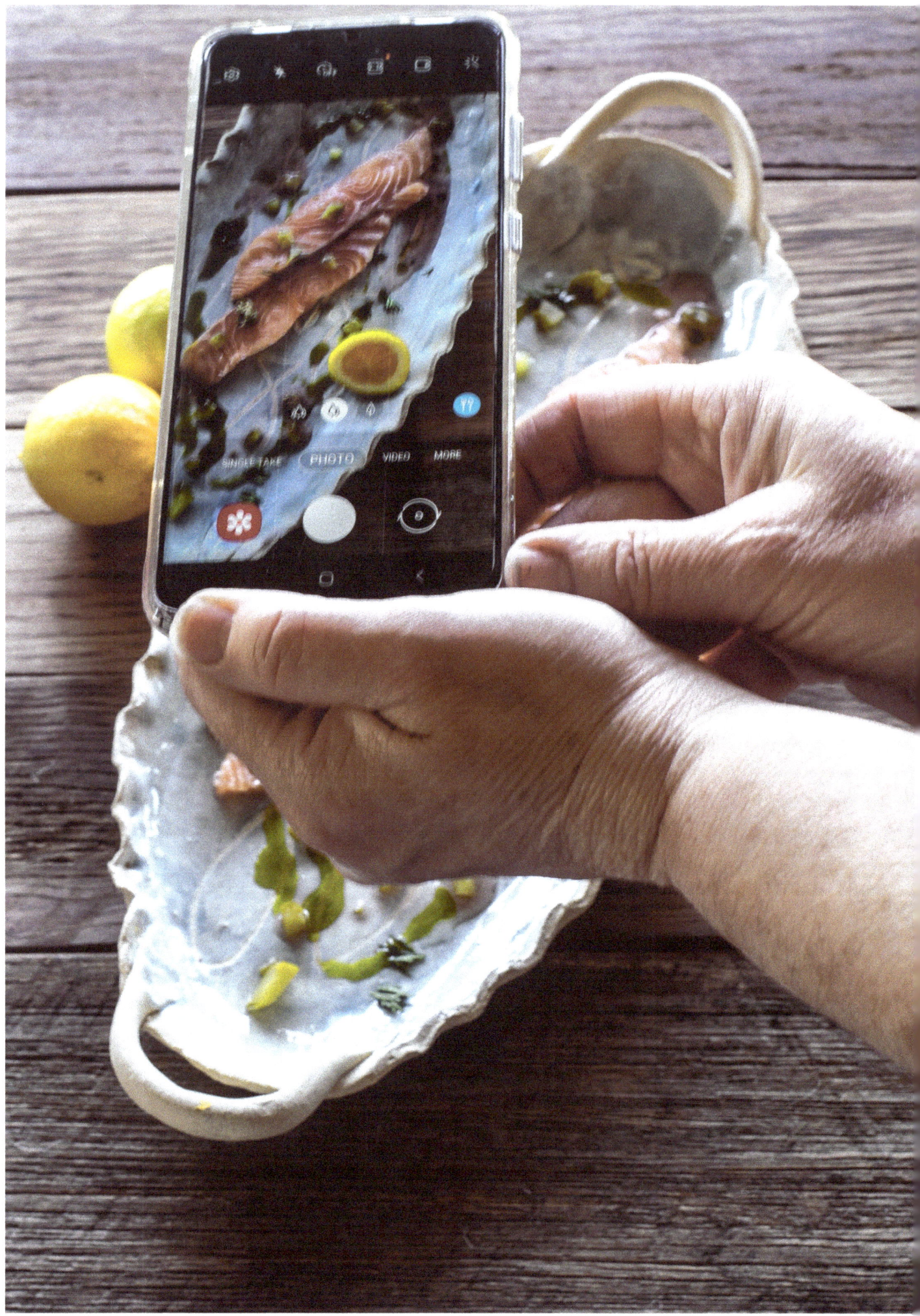

Feeling inspired?
Would you like to learn more?

You might enjoy my many in person and online workshops!

I cover many basics such as:

Seafood Cooking

Bread Making

Photography

Party Planning

Self Publishing

Phone Photography and Food Styling

Please find more information
at www.eloiseemmett.com

Eloise Emmett

CHEF PHOTOGRAPHER STYLIST

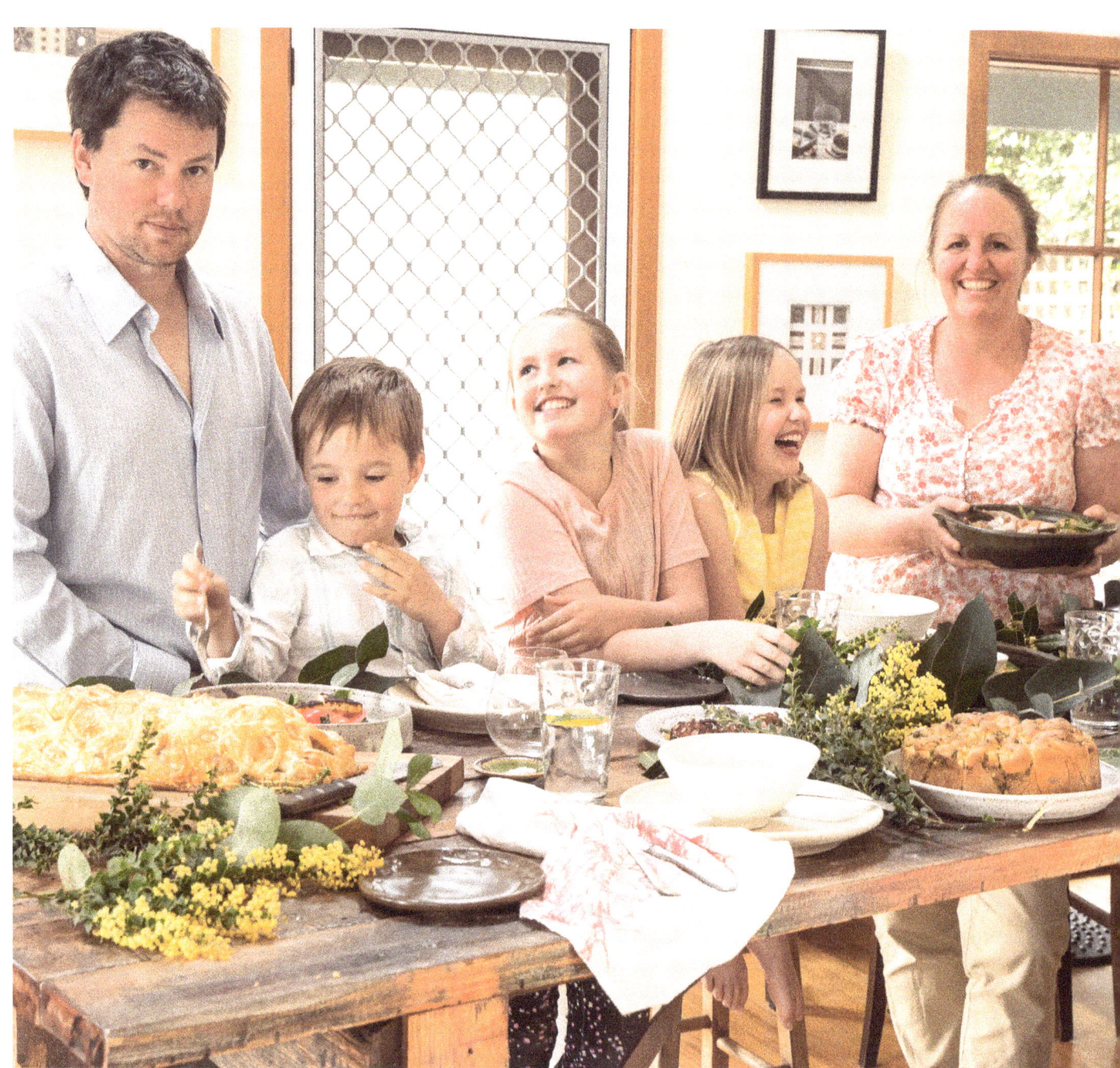

www.ingramcontent.com/pod-product-compliance
Lightning Source LLC
Chambersburg PA
CBHW041622020526
44118CB00052B/2996